SUPER
SWOLE

PUBLISHED BY PUG NINE

A CIP catalogue record for this book is available from the British Library

Pug Nine prefers paper-free publishing whenever possible.

ISBN 978-0-9935288-1-1 *Paper First Edition*

STUDIO 53 • 15 INGESTRE PLACE • SOHO • LONDON • W1F 0DU

WWW.PUGNINE.COM

GETTING SWOLE IS HEALTHY.

BUT STILL,

SEE YOUR DOCTOR BEFORE YOU START.

(NO ONE CAN SEE YOUR GAINS IN A COFFIN)

THE DEFINITION

I know you just want to get on with the training. I salute you. A real man doesn't need instructions! But it might be good to read this quick intro and see where the book is coming from. That way, you'll know if we think the same. And if we do, the journey will be much smoother.

WHY SWOLE?

For some, *swole* might sound weird, new, or even stupid. It means *muscular, jacked, ripped*, or whatever you normally use to describe a body that's in great shape. I could have chosen any word, but *swole* contains emotion. And emotions make us act. Seriously, just imagine that feeling when you take off your shirt and reveal *an amazing physique*. Maybe you can imagine other people watching. Yeah baby, look - at - their - faces - now!

You might be thinking - *so what?* - gyms are full of great bodies. A few gyms are, but the thing is, the world isn't full of people in gyms. In fact most people don't workout. Having a great body is still very rare. It's like walking around with a trophy - and like all trophies - people love to know how it was won.

There will be a few who say looking great means being shallow, but trust me, *none* of these people have ever looked great. If they had, they would instantly realize that the feeling of confidence which comes from owning a physique *is* worth it. If you're smart, you can have an amazing body **and** an amazing life in other areas. Having one doesn't stop the other. They actually *enhance* each other. Being in tip-top condition means that you have to be focused, determined, and generally in the zone.

All of these are mental skills, which once developed, improve other parts of your life.

WHY SUPER?

Again, it's all about emotion. You must feel a buzz to make you take action. Our modern world is a competitive one, with digital media pushing and pulling us all day long. Although being swole is a great start in itself, **being *super* swole is about being ahead of the curve**. This may sound like amateur psychology, but it's genuinely important. If you feel hyped, you are more likely to make the kind of changes which separate you from the chasing pack. Being **super swole** *is* the goal. Leave average behind.

WHY 15 LBS IN SIX WEEKS?

Although human beings vary, **adding 15 pounds of muscle in 6 weeks makes *anyone* look better**. Much better. You'll look better in and out of your clothes. You'll feel *solid* in and out of the gym. And, you'll be *strong* outside and in. That sounds obvious, but being strong becomes subconscious in *everything* you do. Someone strong (and in lean condition), has swagger. And when you have swagger, i.e. confidence, you make smarter decisions. Smarter decisions = happier life.

PLEASE SIR, CAN I HAVE SOME MORE?

You can gain more than 15 pounds of muscle generally, but in 6 weeks, it's a push. So why limit to 6 weeks then? There's an old saying in training, "two months, too long".

If something seems too long, too far away, it saps motivation. Or it can make you slack off and assume there's time to play catch up. Forget slacking right now. Why not just a month? Although it would get you amped, some people spend the first 7 to 10 days finding their feet. This isn't a waste, but it robs us of some precious growth time.

Six weeks is the optimum time span for a new program. It's a period you can "hold" in your thoughts, and give everything you've got.

ANY GAINS WILL DO, RIGHT?

By the way, I'm talking about adding 15 pounds of muscle, not fat, and not water bloat. For most of society, putting on weight means getting chubbier. Adding a bit of muscle and a *lot* of fat is old school. The idea that you bulk up and strip down is a flawed one. Excess body fat is useful in just one sport (long distance swimming at sea). For everyone else, excess body fat will destroy your hormones, and your intensity for life itself.

I CAN SEE RIGHT THROUGH YOU

How can I be so sure about adding muscle? The proof is in the pudding known as DEXA. This is a large, lay-down x-ray machine that tells you how much fat and muscle you have, *to the gram*. Studying this kind of data, I've seen average guys add 15 pounds of muscle in 6 weeks (about 7kg in Europe's metric system, or "a stone" in the UK).

Whatever I say, you will meet guys who'll laugh and tell you it's not possible to gain 15 pounds in a year, and that doing it in 6 weeks is just a dream. Or they might also tell you it is possible, but **only with drugs**. Or **only with enough drugs**. Or **only with tren**. Or **only by being black**. Or **only by being a certain type of black**. Or **only if you're German like Arnold** (he's *Austrian*). Or **only if you're new to training**. Or **only if you're used to training**. Or **only if you're a genetic freak**. Or **only if you're a Hollywood actor with dietitians, a cook, a trainer and drugs**. If you believe these comforting urban myths, you will *only* be insulting your own untested potential.

<u>I've seen natural athletes gain 15 pounds in 6 weeks, time and time again, and they've been from every background possible.</u>

White, Black, Chinese, Indian, Jewish, Muslim or Atheist. Teenagers and those in their 50s. Guys with skinny wrists. Guys with wrists bigger than a skinny guy's *knees*. Hairy chest guys, and guys like Bieber. *Even* Bieber!

Genes make a difference, but they're the start line, not the finish.

Most importantly, and I do mean most importantly:

Anyone can make gains and become a better version of themselves.

KNOWING YOUR LIMITS

How far *your* genes will take you, I can't say. Even the latest DNA testing can't say for sure. **Only you can try to find out**. And even then, you might never actually hit those limits, because humans are born with massive potential for physical and mental improvement. The only certainty is to push hard, as soon as you can, and get close as possible to the perfect image in your head. As you get there, you might find your *ideal-you* changes. You might want more, or you might be happy with what you have. Whatever it is:

You'll only find your limits if you are smart enough to get near them.

And trust me, that's the true gift: the ability to push yourself smart and hard enough to find your limits. In *anything*. You've already proved you're better than 90% of people, by reading this book and therefore investing in your future.

WHAT YOU'LL NEED

Two boxes of tren, one of insulin, a fridge of GH, and a lifetime membership of *Gold's Gym Venice*. Seriously, you need yourself, some weight, some food, and some time. If you've got this book, you've got yourself, and you've decided you've got some time. Does being at a gym help? Absolutely. Is it the only way? Not at all. It's important for you to realize that the human body doesn't know *where* you work out. **Weight is weight, gravity is gravity**. Inside, your body senses many things, but the biggest factors, like weight applied to a muscle and how intensely you work it, come from effort.

Don't bitch if you haven't got a great gym. Change gyms. Get some cash if being where you are feels *not enough*. Start right now to do one thing, **take responsibility**. No one cares about bitching. Even our friends don't. They nod in agreement when we tell them about that annoying thing that just happened, but they've got their own stuff to deal with.

When it comes to gaining muscle fast, you literally must be the boss. If you're running a swole 15/6 program, remember: **it only works if you work**.

FOOD FOR THOUGHT

The final thing you need, after yourself, time and weight, is food. You do need to eat slightly differently if you want to gain muscle fast. Specifically, you'll have to eat more *carefully* than average. The body is desperate to stay the same (it's called *homeostasis*). Having more muscle hanging off your frame means it has to find more calories just to keep going. It makes sense for your body to fight against putting it at greater risk of starvation. But if you persist - if you *beast it* - it will give in, and it will give you whatever you repeatedly demand.

WHERE'S YOUR WHY?

Gaining muscle weight isn't that complicated. But what really helps, is if you know *why* you're using a particular strategy, instead of just following the local gym broscience, *YouTube* video or online forum. Copying others is a human habit, and it works for some emergencies. But after a while it's a risk, because you don't know who you're copying, and whether they've got a clue themselves. Unfortunately most gyms are like this, the blind following the blind. Or more specifically, the smaller guys following the bigger guys.

Study up, try stuff, fine tune.

Those six words can help you succeed in many areas. Let's get started.

THE PLAN

This book will be in 3 sections. The first part will be everything you need to know about training. The second part will be everything you need about nutrition. And the final part will be everything else, things you might have forgotten to ask. Many people try to give training or nutrition percentages based on their importance. For example, you often hear it's "80% diet, 20% training", or the other way round. In reality, everything is important. Because of genes, some people do better than others even with a poor diet, and to some degree, even with bad training. But if you're talking about maximum improvement in a short period of time (e.g. six weeks), **training, diet and attitude all matter**.

You don't have to read the book in order, even though it's in order of importance. Some of you might be knowledgeable in a particular area, and feel you can skip past certain bits. While that's generally fine, some of the training and diet advice is *specific* to *Super Swole*. So, if possible, read the whole thing and in the order it's written.

There may be some of you who are actually quite advanced in training terms, and have picked this up out of curiosity, or perhaps because you need a boost. If that sounds familiar, I say follow this completely and *let go* of your previous ideas. Yep, even if you think you know better. Personal trainers, exercise professors and even Olympic athletes sometimes need to follow the advice of another, simply to kick start their enthusiasm. It can be hard to motivate yourself when you've "seen it all before".

This apparently basic book could actually solve all your complex questions. They say "the devil is in the details". I say "God it's simple".

Finally, to help you make sense of the chapters, each one ends with a little **bro vs pro** summary. The rise of online forums and the *YouTube* fitness community have given rise to the term **broscience**.

This often makes light of the average gym trainee and their ideas. It's mainly stated by those who consider themselves serious "strength athletes".

In reality, in-gym bodybuilding discoveries have actually contributed lots to science, spotting trends *way before* those in lab coats could prove it. Because science journals are easily found online, we all have a tendency to think we're experts, and dismiss gym discoveries as *broscience*. Later research might prove the opposite. So, while a lot of broscience *is* nonsense, it's worth keeping an open mind. We will take on the really rubbish stuff, and balance it up with what I call **proscience**, the more established truths at the current time. Let's give you an example as we close this part out:

BRO VS PRO

bro

×   training is everything
×   diet is everything
×   genes are everything

pro

✓   correct training is important
✓   correct diet is important
✓   determination is more important than your genes

SECTION 1:
IN THE GYM

LET'S SPLIT

Here's the first question you'll be asking, "What kind of routine should I do?". And those who know a bit will add, "How should I split up my body parts?". The simple response is:

To make maximum gains in minimum time, you must use a full-body workout.

To convince you, it's important to take a quick bodybuilding history class. Trust me, it's worth it.

SPLIT ROUTINE 101

Until the mid 60s, <u>every</u> bodybuilder on the planet used a full-body workout. It was popular because they worked, and because they *felt* right. About then, 3 key things changed:

- steroids became available in the US
- bodybuilding magazines became popular
- new types of gym equipment became available

Steroids had been around a few years earlier, but it was only in the 1960s that an average dude could get his hands on some. At that time, we didn't know about side effects, and they were as legal as *Coca-Cola*. Working out was becoming cool and a young entrepreneur called *Joe Weider* spotted the business potential, setting up the first widely available bodybuilding magazines.

Joe realized to inspire people, you needed a hero. In future movie star Arnold Schwarzenegger, he found a genius. Seeing the 19 year old win a physique show in Europe, Joe rushed him over to the US, and set him up in sunny California. The early mags focused on Arnie and a few other dudes who would become the very first competitive bodybuilders.

While this was happening, new gym equipment was being invented. Imagine the world until then, with just barbells, dumbbells, dipping bars, and sometimes not even a flat bench. Along comes Joe Gold (who set up *Gold's Gym*), and Jack La Lanne, the man behind the phrase *No Pain, No Gain... (... take it from La Lanne)*. Suddenly there were lat pulldown machines, leg extensions, and cable crossovers. Training heaven.

Arnie and the other guys would take gear (remember it was legal) and strive to build a detailed body with no weak body parts. To get that, and take advantage of all the amazing new equipment, they logically divided their workouts into parts, or *splits*. This allowed them to zone in on individual areas. On top of all this, working out in a beautiful climate made being in the gym *fun*. Why do 3 days a week when you could do 6.

Slowly but surely, and as promoted by the magazines, everyone was encouraged to split their workouts, and increase their total training volume. Now, there was actually nothing wrong with increasing the volume, as science would go on to prove, even for natural guys. But reducing the **frequency** of how <u>often</u> you hit a muscle was a bad idea, and it still is. Why?

HIT ME BABY ONE MORE TIME

In natural guys, training boosts protein synthesis for 48 hours.

This means for 2 days, your body is increasing the protein content of your muscles, i.e. repairing and making them a bit bigger. Protein and water is literally what your muscles are made of. After a couple of days, protein synthesis goes back to *normal*. That is, you go back to being an Average Joe, roughly balancing the protein that goes into your body, and the protein that leaves. You keep your level of muscle tissue *constant*, repairing your internal organs, building up your lost skin cells, and letting your hair grow. As I can assume you're not just interested having cool hair, it's important to state right now:

Training a body part *less* than once every 4 days is not ideal.

If you follow the broscience, you'll be encouraged to think training a body part once every 5 to 7 days is optimal. It's not, at least in natural guys.

Training a body part once every 5 to 7 days <u>slows down your progress</u>.

If you train on a modern split routine, hitting your body parts with once per week frequency, you'll spend the majority of your week with an Average Joe's physiology. That is, you'll grow for a bit, and then *maintain*. This is a crazy strategy, and if you're looking to get swole in 6 weeks, it's utterly unthinkable.

Even in guys who take gear, it's worth training more often.

Arnold is often criticized for popularizing split routines. The interesting truth is this:

- before coming to America, Arnold used full-body workouts
- Arnold's split routines *still* hit body parts 2 or 3 times per week

Most people don't know about the last point. Arnold generally trained with simple workouts, but in the months leading up to a show, he'd train 6 days per week. Unlike a modern split, which hits a body part once per week, Arnold would train chest separately, but on Monday, Wednesday and Friday. He'd do the same for back, legs and so on. The combination of great genes, high volume / high frequency training, medical grade steroids, and unbeatable determination, made Arnold the legend that still graces the cover of *Flex* magazine *today*.

Somehow between the 1960s and now, split routines grew, but in a different format. As said, training a body part once every 5 to 7 days is now the norm. Full-body workouts are seen only as beginner stuff. Research shows that regardless of opinion, protein synthesis only lasts for around 48 hours. Worrying or exciting new research (depending on what you do now) hints that the more you train, the *shorter* this enhanced period of protein growth lasts. I'll say it simply:

The more training you have under your belt, the more frequency becomes *important*. To keep growing, you must train *more* frequently than most.

It's the opposite of what today's trainers and trainees think. They ignore the research, or don't know about it, or are perhaps scared of full-body workouts. Some fear comes from the thought of answering that classic gym-buddy question:

"What you training today?"

Most guys haven't got the guts to say "everything", even if they instinctively love training full-body. It's safer to fit in with the crowd, and more social to join a buddy and *smash chest on Monday*. But fitting-in is something your body doesn't care about.

For optimal results, you must think independently.

So by now, I hope you're beginning to realize that full-body workouts are the only way to go. They will help you get to your goal *quicker*, and that itself is crucial for two reasons:

- motivation is highest when a goal can be achieved faster
- hormones gradually lower with age, so use them quickly

There are also practical reasons to push full-body training. If you miss a workout, you simply hit the gym when your schedule gets back on track. Everything is treated equally. If you miss a body part split, it pushes your whole regime out of sync.

TOTAL RECOVERY

Full-body workouts also allow the body *in general* to recover faster, and more completely.

With training frequencies of more than about 3 times per week, your immunity can be lowered. Getting a cold or infection sucks, and nothing stops progress faster than being ill. Mentally, hitting the gym too often via split routines can literally become *routine*, i.e. boring. Spending too much time travelling back and forth gets draining. If you're addicted to breaking gym attendance records, you could be avoiding something else in your life. It's smarter to sort that out instead.

There is also some new evidence that training smaller body parts, like biceps, around the same time that you train bigger bits, like legs, makes the smaller ones *grow faster*. If you train with a full-body workout, you'll hit everything together, and maximize this effect. If you use a split routine, only some of your body parts can get this boost.

BUT FULL-BODY WORKOUTS ARE TOO TIRING

Really?

Man up!

Seriously, if you haven't got the fitness to carry out a full-body workout, something's wrong, either physically or mentally. Yes, *in the beginning* you might find them tough, especially if you're used to training under the broscience 45-minute time limit. Bro legend states that if you go a second over 45 minutes, your testosterone will drop, and you'll shrivel up like a raisin.

There is no truth in that.

THE RISE AND FALL OF A MYTH

We now understand that hormones which rise and fall *around* a workout, like testosterone and cortisol, change so quickly back to normal, that their levels <u>don't</u> affect your progress.

Your *average* levels of testosterone make a difference (you want them high), and your *average* levels of cortisol matter also (you want those low). So, ditch the idea that a long full-body workout will destroy your gonads. It won't. Instead, focus on stimulating maximum growth by inducing some serious damage.

BUT WHAT ABOUT MY UPPER CHEST?

Today's biggest concern about doing a full-body workout seems to be that it won't let you develop a balanced body. In theory, if you put all your favorite exercises for each body part into one massive full-body workout, you'd be in the gym all day.

So you need to specialize, right? That's what broscience suggests. For example, if you want a thick slab of upper pec, the only way to is to hit incline after incline. This sounds logical. But it's BS for two reasons.

- most exercises are very similar to other exercises
- a muscle's shape changes most when you make it bigger

Your genes are your genes, and in terms of an individual muscle's shape, you can't redesign it.

You can *slightly* emphasize different bits of the biggest body part groups, like legs, chest and back. But slightly.

The fastest way to a balanced body is actually to make your muscles bigger.

Flat benching for example, doesn't just hit the middle of the pec. It hits 90% of it. And if you ever look at an elite powerlifter (in shape) who mainly does flat bench, they will have good pecs from top to bottom. Certainly way more than the average gym dude who has done thousands more sets of incline. The difference is due to the overall *size* of the muscle, and being lean enough to see it all. This last point is important.

Excess body fat hides the body's *natural* symmetry. When you get leaner, you will notice that all your muscle groups look much more even. Fat around the pecs is usually around the lower and outer pecs, making them look gorilla-like in some people. That's just where fat tends to store in most guys. As you strip it off, they will appear more like an even slab.

In terms of exercises being like most other exercises, it's amazing how unknown this fact is. And it is a **fact**. A flat barbell bench press is almost identical to a flat dumbbell bench press. Yes, they feel different, but they both pull the arms from out to the side, to over the mid-line of the chest (technically known as *horizontal adduction of the humerus*). The dumbbells pull more naturally in this case, and are generally the better exercise. Doing both might be fun, but the time wasted in switching set-ups *is* time wasted. And, doing both would be a waste of physical effort compared to just nailing more sets of dumbbell bench.

This book cannot give you all the anatomy skills to work out which exercises are the same as each other, but I will list recommended and not recommended ones. It's up to you to study others, and discover why many routines are full of fluff, i.e. duplicate movements.

You need to pick the best exercises, and hit them hard.

FREQUENTLY ASKED QUESTION

So to summarize the frequency question, in terms of *Super Swole*, here it is.

You must do a full-body workout - <u>at least</u> - once every 3 days.

And:

You must do a full-body workout - <u>at most</u> - every other day.

For example, you'll work out like this:

EVERY OTHER DAY (HIGHEST FREQUENCY)

Monday
Wednesday
Friday
Sunday
Tuesday
Thursday
Saturday

keep repeating

or

FIXED DAYS PER WEEK (MEDIUM FREQUENCY)

Monday, Wednesday, Friday
Tuesday, Thursday, Saturday
Wednesday, Friday, Sunday
Thursday, Saturday, Monday
Friday, Sunday, Tuesday
Saturday, Monday, Wednesday
Sunday, Tuesday, Thursday

or

EVERY THIRD DAY (LOWEST FREQUENCY)

Monday, Thursday, Sunday, Wednesday, Saturday, Tuesday, Friday, etc.

Some people prefer fixed days because it fits the rest of their schedule, or gym opening times. Others like the variety of training on different days. Or, it's as simple as you use the frequency that works best for you physically.

You may find that with more training, you recover quicker. Be prepared to shift your routine slightly if you notice this.

So, during *Super Swole*, you'll have somewhere between 14 and 21 workouts. How will you know what's best for you? A simple guide is if you *feel* ready to go and *clear* in your mind, have a workout. If you have *slight* soreness, you can still train. Soreness tends to occur after switching to a new routine, or new movement pattern, i.e. dramatically different exercise. Although this sounds unscientific, I'm afraid this is where science runs out slightly, and the *art of training* takes over. Yes I know, it sounds lame, but it's actually true in this case. Fine-tuning your workout frequency might take a while, but eventually, you'll know what works best for your particular body.

Long after this book, you may reduce your training frequency to once every 4 days, roughly twice per week. Remember, that's for those interesting in adding more muscle. A mere 90 workouts per year. But if you don't mind *maintaining*, i.e. that's not growing, but keeping what you have, then you could do that by hitting 'parts once every 5 to 7 days. If you still like the full-body workout feeling, this means **you could literally maintain all your muscle with one full-body workout per week**. I have witnessed people perfectly maintain lots of muscle with doing exactly that. The intensity has to be quite high, but this comes naturally with only one workout per week. It's also a useful thing to know if you haven't quite finished reaching your muscle goals, but need some downtime to get on with other stuff. Simply crank it back up once you're ready to go again.

SICK WORKOUT BRO

This is a special note for those who get ill. If you are sick *above* the neck, e.g. a head cold, you can still train. If you are sick *below* the neck, e.g. chest infection, it's best to rest. All stress - *and training is a form of stress* - hits the immune system, squashing it down for a few hours after training. It does this by temporarily damaging the delicate lining of your gut (alcohol, excess heat stress and smoking do this too). If you're already ill, this could keep you ill for longer than normal. While we're here, **look after your personal hygiene in the 2 hours immediately after training**. This is when your immune system is at its lowest. Gyms can be dirty places, even home gyms. If you don't shower, at least wash your hands *carefully* with soap (tops of hands too, and above the wrist bone, keeping the action going when rinsing), and <u>avoid</u> sick people if possible. Sound like boring advice? Nothing's more boring than being sick and unable to train. Dude, use that soap!

IT'S ALL ABOUT THE BIKE

It's worth pointing out a couple of extra things here. **Excess duration cardio, like cycling or running does reduce *average* testosterone levels**. More than 30 miles per week of jogging can turn a young dude's hormones into his granddad's. Long duration cardio can also increase *average* cortisol levels. So, beware. More on cardio later.

TIME TO GIVE UP

Research also shows that longer workout sessions *of any kind* tend to make people quit. So when you get down to training, don't hang around beyond the training itself or you could get bored, resent working out and quit completely.

After about 2 weeks of doing full-bodys, you should be adjusted fine. If people pass comments about how long your session is, politely ignore them. There's nothing cool about being in and out of the gym fast if you haven't stimulated much growth. If you must answer, remind them that overall, you'll spend less total time in reaching your goals. By then, you can maintain with less training if you want.

This has been a massive chapter, because it's massively important. There's stuff in the next few about what exercises to choose, and others on sets and reps. Before we go *bro vs pro*, I'll sum up the main point in one line:

You must use a full-body workout to get swole fast.

BRO VS PRO

bro

- × full-body workouts are for beginners only
- × full-body workouts are too tiring for experienced guys
- × full-body workouts are useless for developing a balanced body

pro

- ✓ full-body workouts are for beginners to Olympic champions
- ✓ full-body workouts force you to train with smart efficiency
- ✓ full-body workouts maximize mass, shape and overall health

WARMING UP

Before you even consider sets and reps, consider what makes your muscles happy. Muscles work best when they're warm. Not hot, just warm. They increase temperature when you move them, mainly because your blood flows *through* them. Blood is warm. It's like a hairdryer, and your muscles are like elastic bands. When muscles are at their *optimal* temperature, they contract *harder*, and are less likely to get injured. What's the best way to warm up?

TIME OF DAY

Strictly speaking, this bit isn't a "technique", but an observation that naturally helps you "warm-up". Your body is cooler when you wake, and gradually gets warmer throughout the day. Studies find that strength is highest from late afternoon to early evening. By this time, you're likely to have eaten a few meals, further increasing the chance of feeling strong. It might not literally be the time of day itself, with more detailed research revealing it takes about 6 to 7 hours after you *wake up* to reach a peak. Of course, not everyone's the same, and for years I relied on the research to *tell* people when they would feel best. And eventually, some brave souls told me I was wrong.

With genetic testing, it now appears some humans really are suited to the morning (so-called "larks"), while some seem happiest at night (so-called "owls"). Follow-up studies tested performance, usually in intellectual tests, but also some light-physical activities too.

Because hitting the weights is affected by your mental focus, I suggest the following:

Train at the time you feel your best.

I am aware that for some people, feeling their best clashes when they're busy with something else (e.g. their partner, work crashing-out time). Still, if you happen to discover that definite time zone when you feel great (energized, itching "to do"), try having a workout. It's the ultimate first step of a "warm-up".

GENERAL SYSTEM WARM-UP

Warming up your *whole* body is a smart thing. It sends a strong message to *all* interrelated systems (heart, lungs, kidneys, liver etc.) about what you're going to do. A warm-up of this kind doesn't take long. In fact, it takes about 3 minutes. Sport scientists call reaching a good temperature and where everything flows, *steady state*. If you're working out in a gym, and have access to a treadmill, use it. Just walk for three minutes. That's it. The next best thing would be you actually walking *in the real world* on your way to the gym. If you train at home, go outside and walk for a few minutes. Literally, just 3 minutes.

To warm up, excessive cardio is not necessary, and can drain you. Just walking at a normal speed for 3 minutes is enough.

If you can't use a treadmill, use what you can, e.g. an elliptical trainer or stationary exercise bike. Even walking *around* the gym will help. So what if people stare.

Apart from a general warm-up, you need to warm up for your actual sets. I'll cover that in a separate bit. Oh, one more thing.

STRETCHING THE TRUTH

Do not stretch before your workout.

Muscles have strength because tiny sensors inside them that know when they're being stretched. Pull your arm out to the side, and it wants to spring back to the middle. Jump on a basketball court and your knees will slightly bend before you push upwards. This tension and release is called the *stretch-reflex*, and it not only helps you copy Michael Jordan, but it keeps your skeleton upright when choosing which of his boots to buy. It's how we're designed.

If you stretch, no matter how cool you think it looks, you're detraining the natural stretch-reflex. Stretch your pecs for 5 minutes and then pull your arm out to the side in the way I mentioned before. It will spring back to the middle, but with less tension. Here's the simple truth, broken down in bold:

Stretching before a workout reduces strength and power. Even stretching one hour before has been shown to decrease performance.

You want your strength and power to be optimal, as that's what stimulates growth. But doesn't stretching prevent injury? Not necessarily. And *often*, it causes it. When you hit the weights, you will do the best kind of warm-up and stretch, i.e. one that's made for *that* movement, with the optimal range. This doesn't reduce power or strength. In fact, it improves it. For now, put the hard iron before the soft yoga mat and foam roller.

BRO VS PRO

bro

×   you need to sweat hard as a warm up
×   the time you train makes no difference
×   you should stretch before you workout

pro

✓   a 3 min. general warm-up is optimal for muscle temperature
✓   train at a time when you feel your strongest
✓   do not stretch before your workout

THE JOY OF SETS

In this section, I'm going to cover two areas many trainees often worry about out. How many *sets* should I do? And, how many *reps*.

SETS

When it comes to sets, there are two training styles:

- High *volume*
- High-*intensity*

Both camps agree on one thing: you can train hard, or you can train lots, but you can't do both. I disagree, and so does your body. Let's take a look at each and see what they offer.

HIGH-INTENSITY

Originally promoted by Arthur Jones, the inventor of *Nautilus* gym equipment, high-intensity training believes you must train with serious effort, get the job done, and go home. Specifically, Arthur believed that you could do the job with just one or two sets. He said that on *no* occasion, should someone do more than 3. All kinds of cute analogies were used to make a point, like if you shoot a man dead, why shoot him again. As I said, cute, but not relevant.

High-intensity training does encourage something great: proper effort and on fewer movements (Jones liked full-body workouts only). We now realize that sets taken to *positive failure* - that's when you can't push or pull any more - regardless of weight (up to 30 reps), trigger muscle growth. Because high-intensity uses so few sets, it helps push you closer to this point.

The problems with high-intensity training are injury and motivation. Consistently putting yourself under pressure to nail the perfect all-out set, means you will inevitably use very heavy weights. Using these exclusively - without gradual warm ups - can increase injury risk. 6 times Mr Olympia *Dorian Yates* used a form of high-intensity training throughout his career. Towards the latter end of his Olympia run, he was injured often. It's hard to say whether this was all down to high-intensity work, but it's a possibility.

Also, with the weight always high, the mind-muscle connection tends to be poor. You get strong with high intensity, low-set training, but often muscle growth is slower to progress. And sometimes, the muscles which do grow *aren't* those you intended. They naturally get involved when the weight is so high.

The motivation required for all-out effort in just one or two sets is also a problem. Beginners have a tough time getting that psyched and being able to hit the required intensity. As you get more experienced, you can push harder, but it still takes a certain mindset to enjoy "fighting" in the gym.

In short, high-intensity training isn't much fun. I'm not trying to be down on it, because as mentioned, it has benefits. It encourages someone to carefully select good exercises, and avoid pointless versions of the same movement. And, it pushes the intensity *in the right direction*. For now, let's move on to the other style.

HIGH VOLUME

This is about doing multiple sets, or multiple exercises, perhaps 20 to 30 per body part. It came around at the time of split training, which makes sense. If you're only going to hit a muscle once a week, you better hit it hard. The problem is that you can't combine it with anything other than split training. It just won't go with a full-body workout, and we *need* those frequent workouts to optimize muscle protein stimulation.

Most modern drug using bodybuilders use a high volume approach, but they also work with a reduced frequency, i.e. they hit muscles once every 5 to 7 days. For years, natural bodybuilders have been told to avoid copying their chemically assisted buddies. In fact they did listen, but in the worst way possible. They dropped their sets per exercise and reduced their frequency of hitting body parts to once per week. Ironically, the correct advice is to do *more* training (frequency), not less. A bodybuilder on gear has a permanently elevated testosterone level, which makes *more growth* easier on *less training*.

The good thing about high volume training is that it can encourage a strong mind-muscle connection. This is crucial for building the muscles you want to build, and to reduce injury. Of course, there is a different kind of injury risk - overuse injury - from doing *too* much in total.

WHAT THE RESEARCH SAYS

This is important. Today's sport science has shown some interesting patterns. In an absolute beginner, doing 1 or 3 sets doesn't initially make much difference.

This is because the main improvements come from their nervous system "learning" how to perform exercises more efficiently. In that case, just a single set will do the job.

Our brain is a fast learner on minimal information (i.e. giving it just one set). But over time, doing multiple sets - 3 or more - improves the rate of progress. That is:

Higher set volumes cause more muscle growth, and more strength gains.

The research is very clear on this. Greater numbers of sets obviously send a *greater signal* to the body's muscle machinery (the DNA in each muscle cell), telling it to wake up and adapt fast, i.e. grow. The *metabolic stress* of multiple sets - that's changes in chemicals like lactic acid - is higher the more sets you do. We know for example, that lactic acid triggers growth hormone, the body's most powerful hormone overall. This could benefit muscle growth long-term. Finally, the more times you *mechanically damage* a muscle, especially through repeatedly lengthening the muscle under strain (eccentric contraction), the more you stimulate it to adapt (get bigger).

So where does that leave us? We need to find the best of both worlds, combining high enough intensity with high enough volume, but not too much that we can't do it with a full-body workout. Remember, we need the full-body workout to do all the good stuff *as often as possible*. That means picking a *select* number of exercises, and working them for a moderately high number of sets. First off, how many exercises?

EXERCISE CHOICE

Here's the thing:

Most trainees do too many exercises per body part.

Forget about sets for a moment. I'm talking about doing too many *exercises*, with each one offering hardly any variation from the others. Their incline bench and flat bench end up looking much the same. Their front squats and back squats hit mostly the same muscle tissue. And their variations in curls are simply embarrassing. There is little point in designing your workout like this, other than for the sake of variety. Personal trainers use complicated routines because they know it prevents their clients working out without them. Smart business, silly training.

By picking multiple exercises for the same body part, you risk never finding out which is the most effective one.

It's a Catch-22 with some guys, who often become scared of giving up exercises for fear of getting smaller without them. Although we plan to use a relatively high volume of sets, there's no point in putting your joints through unnecessary stress.

PLANE JANE

Some body parts, like chest, back and thighs can technically tolerate more than one exercise. It's because they are complex muscles, with distinctly different movement patterns, also known as "planes". For example your lats can pull from above, like a pulldown, and from in front, like a seated row. These are genuinely different, with different *nerves* being activated during the rep. This variation in "wiring" suggests that Mother Nature regards them as specialized functions. In such areas, there is a case for variety, but you don't have to hit all angles all the time. Instead of giving them multiple exercises, we can instead give them a few more extra sets than other smaller body parts.

In the three most powerful and natural planes (directions) that the body moves, there's a lot of muscle growth to be had. That's:

1)   Pushing forwards to slightly down (chest movements)
2)   Pulling backwards from slightly above (back movements)
3)   Driving the legs away from the body (thigh movements)

The overhead pushing plane is actually quite weak, and our shoulder is clearly designed for mobility rather than strength. It has ligaments, but is mainly held in place by layers of muscle, including the delts, and the often-injured rotator cuff (4 different muscles). Extremely heavy overhead presses can only build shoulders, triceps and the uppermost part of the chest. These are relatively small areas of muscle mass. If an overhead load is very heavy, we naturally lean back to use the *whole* chest, and we might use the legs too. The overhead press used to be one of *four* tested powerlifting movements, until competitors began to lean so far back, it literally became a low incline press without a bench! It was then removed from competitions (leaving the deadlift, squat and bench).

So, as we'll see in a minute, we'll give these key directions more sets. The smaller muscles happen to be those which already get used in those major three directions, so they need fewer sets. Some hardcore "hardgainer" type trainers suggest not using *any* direct movements for arms or even shoulders. This is a crazy strategy, and proven crazy by new research.

In carefully controlled studies, when training routines get <u>direct</u> arm work, they far outpace those who get none. Some studies find a big increase, some a smaller increase, but all find *an increase*. And I'm sure you'd like your arms and shoulders to not fall behind. You're going to hit them anyway, so best make it official! Let's get back to the key point so far:

The biggest gains come from working a few carefully selected exercises, for moderately high sets, as often as you can.

Therefore, I suggest you:

Use one main exercise per body part during a training cycle.

A training "cycle" is just a fancy term for time spent on a particular program. For example, these 6 weeks during *Super Swole* are a training cycle. Now, you can change exercises for a particular body part eventually, but when should you do that?

CHANGING EXERCISES

You need to change exercises mainly to keep motivation high. Scientifically, there's no evidence to say that doing the same exercise again and again "bores" the body. As long as it's a good exercise, i.e. technically safe, you can keep using it for as long as you like.

The body will continue to adapt and grow as long as you increase weights over time.

But reality shows it can bore *your* mind. As mentioned before, coaches and trainers often change their client's exercises. They know how boredom is just around the corner, which can lead to a loss of training interest (and a loss of pay check).

Put at its simplest, **your body never gets bored, but your mind might**. So, assuming you want to slightly change the muscle hitting emphasis of certain body parts (e.g. legs, back and chest), how often should you switch up? Here's the rub:

If you want to change exercises, do it a *maximum* of 4 times per year, i.e. <u>at most, once every three months</u>.

If you do it more often, it becomes very difficult to assess your progress. If you find yourself addicted to changing exercises, be honest; perhaps you're scared of putting in the effort. Okay, let's get back to the more important *number of sets* issue. How many do you need?

To get swole, you need to complete 6 sets per major plane (chest, back, thighs) and 3 sets for minor muscle groups (biceps, triceps, shoulders).

This includes warm-ups. Studies have shown that up to 8 sets are very effective for increasing strength, and with increased strength, increased size eventually follows. It follows even more if these sessions are performed with frequency, which is what *Super Swole* is all about. But, 8 are too many for our needs, and would tip the frequent full-body workout slightly over the top. Eight sets would also mean you'd select slightly lower weights, and this would reduce overall gains. For those who worry about their smaller muscle groups like biceps and triceps - *relax* - because they do relatively better *in* a full-body routine, getting heavy indirect work from major back and chest movements.

So, how should you perform these multiple sets?

SET STYLE

Muscles work hardest when they're:

- warm
- prepared for a specific movement

A general warm-up is good when you start at the gym. It sends blood around the body, increases the heart rate making it ready for action, and generally brings you to an optimal working temperature. This literally takes just a few minutes, e.g. that 3-minute walk on a treadmill. For a specific warm-up, you need to perform *warm-up sets*. When you do a light set of a movement, the <u>specific</u> nerves required to electrify and contract <u>those</u> muscles get brought to life. The more you work the desired muscles, the more your nervous system lights up. And like most things in the body, *gradual* is best. This is why I promote use of a **pyramid set style**. It's old fashioned, it's instinctive, and it still works better than anything else.

PYRAMID STYLE

It's probably how you train already. You start light, and gradually get heavier. That's the nuts and bolts of it. As you get heavier, the reps may drop. With your heaviest sets coming later, you will benefit from these factors:

- increased local muscle temperature
- enhanced nerve firing
- superior mind-muscle connection
- widest selection of muscle fibers hit

Don't worry about the last point, all will make sense soon. For now, know that starting light and *gradually* adding weight, is the smartest way to train. It builds confidence with each set, and due to the gradually increased heat, nerve firing and enhanced mind-muscle connection, you really hit the targeted muscle *hard*. The lighter sets are metabolically stressful (they change the chemical world in and around your muscle tissue, helping growth), and the heavier sets are mechanically damaging (also forcing muscles to protect their future by getting bigger). It's an ideal way to train. Let's move onto reps.

REP RANGE

There really is a wide range of reps that build muscle. We used to think some muscles, like legs, needed higher reps. Often the unscientific reason given, "it's a bigger muscle". We also used to believe that certain muscles, due to having different types of fibers - fast or slow twitch - needed a different approach. Fast twitch fibers, as the name suggests, contract fast and generate lots of power. Slow twitch fibers contract slower, but have good endurance. In most people, their calf muscles are slow twitch, and their nearby hamstrings, fast. But generally, it's very difficult to tell. Even genetic testing can't tell you about your whole body, i.e. every *individual* muscle. To truly define muscle fiber type, you'd have to extract tissue and study it under a microscope. It's a painful process that's normally used on quads. Good luck doing it on your forearms.

FULL RANGE

We now know that everyone can work their entire *range of fibers*, if they work a *range of reps*. Now, I'm not talking about anything beyond **ten**. That's right, 10.

And of course, you can't go less than 1 rep (well, that's called "HELP!"). By using a pyramid system, starting light, and gradually adding weight, you can hit the vast majority of your fibers. You won't hit many of the **Type 1** fibers, the true *endurance* types. They don't grow much anyway. But you will hit those called **Type 2A** (*intermediate*), and **Type 2B** (*fast*). Both these fibers grow. The type 2B will only grow with the heavier, later sets, possibly only the last few reps.

Sprinters tend to have much more type 2B than bodybuilders, who are made mainly of type 2A. Type 2B grow with the highest tension, like sprinting itself, and truly heavy loads (which sprinters tend to use when hitting the gym).

Ten rep sets aren't too long, which keeps focus and technique high. Beyond 10 reps takes too long, and as most people aren't truly working near their maximum, longer sets are too light. They also raise lactic acid levels excessively, which causes muscle failure due to pain (quite good for growth), rather than mechanical exhaustion (even better).

What should your *heaviest* set be, in terms of reps? It's okay to go down to 4 reps fairly regularly, and sometimes, even see what you can do for a 1-rep max (maximum). You need to be supervised by someone to do this safely. Does a 1-rep max build muscle? Not *directly*. But it sets the stage for more strength, translating to greater numbers of heavier reps in future workouts.

Generally aim to work between 4 and 10 reps, but don't panic if you fall outside of this range.

When you can easily sail past 10, make a note to increase the weight next time.

CHRISTMAS TREE

I said pyramid before, and I lied, sort of. Our reps follow more of a *Christmas tree* shape. I shall explain:

First set

Instead of starting with 10 reps, *always* stop at 5. I know you can do more! The weight's light. But you do *not* want to waste any energy on this first set, beyond preparing your nervous system to work better. It's common to walk into a gym and see a guy who's capable of benching 3 plates a side, warming up with just the empty bar. This is about 15% of maximum. Banging out 30 lightning-fast reps is pointless. You activate the nervous system fine, but you also trigger excessive lactic acid, and waste muscle glycogen.

Later on sets will suffer, even if you can't see the connection by then. **Lactic acid reduces the ability of nerves to fire**. Your heavier lifts suffer. So:

Your first set should be at least half, and up to three-quarters of your expected last (heaviest) set. And, STOP at 5 reps. That's 50 to 75%, for 5 reps only.

This will warm you up nicely for more. The second set will have a strong mind-muscle connection after doing this careful warm-up, and you won't have put your technique or strength at risk by raising lactic acid. This low-rep first set is the plant pot shaped base of our Christmas tree. Ah ha! Yep, you get it.

Each set beyond the first, you add weight. You will either use jumps dictated by going up in dumbbell sizes, or by adding plates to the bar / machine stack. It's impossible to give numbers here, as it varies from exercise to exercise, and also with time.

Increase the weight each set, enough to encourage you to drop a rep or two.

As you "climb the tree", the reps will be lowered. None of these sets should be taken to failure, i.e. to where you can't move. It's not necessary, especially with our combined volume and frequency of training. But still:

You should aim to be *uncomfortable* at the end of each work set. It's the point where your technique starts to get *shaky*.

If you *are* capable of more than 10 reps, don't just stop. Always use the *uncomfortable* point as your guide, and **increase the weight next time**, perhaps a bit more for all that exercise's sets. Normally, as you get a few sets in, you should be heading down to hitting around 5 or 6 reps.

THE FINAL SET

This actually gets its own section (coming up), but for now, you can appreciate it will be your heaviest set.

After gradually increasing the weight, you will have a strong mind-muscle connection, good pump - and crucially - you should be *mentally* warmed-up for the final set push.

The last set should be tough, but still enjoyable.

As I said, there's a bit more about the last set coming up.

REST TIME BETWEEN SETS

It's important to neither rush nor dawdle in the gym. We used to think that fast training boosted testosterone and growth hormone. It can do, but the hormone boost is so short-lived, it makes no difference to muscle growth. Rushing can make a difference to your tiredness though, leaving you exhausted with relatively rubbish numbers. Resting for too long can make your muscles cool slightly, and as the body perceives the *threat* of another assault (set) has gone, it reduces its strength potential. The nerves calm down, and you lose their electrical boost. So what is the optimal amount of rest between sets?

THE CHEMICAL BROTHERS

ATP, the energy molecule, and its little bro CP (creatine phosphate), recover:

50% within 30 seconds
75% within 1 minute
90% within 2 minutes
98% within 3 minutes

Considering this data, and practical gym research:

Rests between sets should be between 1 and 2 minutes. Use a timer in the beginning, until you get an instinct for what's good.

The rest after your first set (i.e. warm-up set) only has to be 1 minute. The weight would have been light, and not taxed your ATP energy system. <u>Do rest for the whole minute though</u>, as too quick a rest will spark the dogs of lactic acid into life, and once they growl at you, they might stay for the whole workout (reducing strength, mind-muscle connection, and motivation).

If you're going for an all-out last set, give yourself up to 3 minutes before you hit it. But not more. Only powerlifters can benefit from beyond the third minute. Let's repeat the message so you really absorb the concept:

Rest long enough to lift strong and tear up your muscle, but be quick enough to chemically damage it too. Rest 1 to 2 minutes.

A mental analogy is waves hitting the beach, with the sea being your training, and the beach, your muscle. The waves are heavy reps lashing against your muscle, breaking it down. And the seawater is a chemical stress, washing over them and continuing the job. Finally, visiting the beach often is your analogy for frequently working out and with enough volume.

The entire workout should take around 90 to 120 minutes. As I stated earlier, expect others to criticize this amount. And rest assured, just because you go beyond 45 minutes, you won't turn into a pumpkin. Here's a summary of what we've covered:

- Do one exercise per body part
- Use 6 sets per major exercise direction, 3 for minors
- Rest 1 to 2 minutes between most sets
- The first set is a 5-rep warm-up
- Every set beyond is 10 reps or less (add weight when 10's easy)
- Add weight each set, dropping a rep or two as needed
- The last set will be your heaviest
- Change exercises at most once every 12 weeks

BRO VS PRO

bro

×   high volume is good / bad
×   high intensity is good / bad
×   multiple exercises are necessary

pro

✓   a combo of higher volume and intensity is optimal
✓   one exercise per 'part helps you focus on improving
✓   6 sets of 4 - 10 on major planes hits most fibers for growth

FAIL TO SUCCEED

There is much written about the importance of taking sets to exhaustion, what's technically known as **training to failure**. Some of it's broscience, some of it *is* science, and some of it takes reality into account. In the 1960s, training to failure was promoted by Arthur Jones, the guy who invented *Nautilus* branded machines. He was a brilliant man (like his son Gary, who invented *Hammer Strength*), who believed in full-body workouts and training to failure, often with one set only (three at most). But, at that time, sport science was in its childhood, and Arthur simply didn't have access to the studies we have today. While many of his thoughts about exercise choice and full-body workouts are still correct, we now have evidence that higher volume training grows more muscle.

1993 A.D. (AFTER DORIAN)

In later years, bodybuilding legend Dorian Yates rekindled an interest in *high-intensity training*. When Dorian appeared in 1992, winning his first Mr Olympia, he was scary. When he won his second in '93, the transformation was utterly shocking. Never before or since did a bodybuilder progress *so* much in one year. His freaky level of muscle *combined* with equally freaky conditioning changed bodybuilding forever. Dorian attributed much of his success to training to failure. What most don't realize is that Dorian wasn't a one set guy. He did multiple exercises and warm-ups that would look like regular work-sets to most observers. True enough, he did one genuinely exhausting set-to-failure at the end of each exercise, something we'll touch on in a bit. To see Dorian at his peak, you'll need to *YouTube* him or find a copy of his *Blood and Guts* training tape.

For those who assume this was down to drugs, remember that Dorian had no more than other builders and no better equipment. All he had was his intelligence, genes, and brutal all-out effort on those final sets.

CAN YOU GROW WITHOUT FAILING?

Yes. The volume of sets and reps you use on a particular exercise is your biggest influence on growth. It's also about the load (the weight), and it's slightly about the metabolic stress (how much chemical damage you bring in a certain period of time). Even if you never go to failure, you can grow, and grow quite fast. This assumes that you workout with enough frequency of course. But could you grow *faster* by hitting failure?

Possibly. Some research has shown that to a degree, even light weights - for a set *to failure* around 30 reps - can stimulate growth like a much heavier set. In unscientific terms, it's as if the body views failure as a threat to its safety, and makes muscles bigger to protect their future. Make no mistake, this *is* exciting research. But, as always, research conducted during carefully controlled experiments doesn't mean achieving the same result in your *real* world.

Training to failure has a couple of obvious problems. If you train home alone and are using a barbell bench press, getting stuck under it is no joke. **There are 6 deaths per year in the US from this kind of accident**. Even with dumbbells, going to failure can be risky, especially if you try to lower them *too* carefully, and rip your shoulder joint to pieces.

Also, training to failure beyond about 6 reps, results in large levels of pain. This is usually **lactic acid**. Lactic acid forms when you can't power your body with oxygen quickly enough, and instead switches to internally stored carbs called **glycogen**. This is a *limited* emergency resource that the body tries to save.

The lactic acid makes your muscle and surrounding blood acidic, reducing the electrical transmission of nerve signals. This reduces your power quickly. If you continue beyond the pain threshold, the blood's acidity can make you vomit.

With your nerve electricity not flowing well, co-ordination and technique goes out of the window. On some exercises, poor technique for a short part of the set, i.e. **cheating**, won't be dangerous. But if your technique goes badly wrong on a deadlift or shoulder press, you could do some serious damage. Having said this, don't be fooled into thinking it's always the last reps of a set that does damage. In fact, it's generally the opposite.

Most gym injuries occur on the *first* few reps of a set, when the muscles are at their freshest.

Watch a powerlifting, weightlifting or strongman competition, and you'll see this is the case. Or *YouTube* "muscle tears" and see how often they occur *as* the set starts. Of course, it's not the first rep itself that's damaging, as damage has to build up from time before.

Let's get back to lactic acid. We know that it has some benefits, like triggering growth hormone production. Whether this makes a difference long-term, we don't know for certain. It may be like testosterone and cortisol, rising and falling too quick for the body to notice. If it does have an effect, growth hormone is likely to boost connective tissue like tendons (they join muscle to bone) and ligaments (they join bone to bone). It also reduces body fat, improves skin thickness, and slightly boosts muscle growth. Also, if you're feeling lactic acid, it means you're emptying out those internal stores of carbs, i.e. **glycogen**. In general health terms, this is a cool thing.

Scientists are now discovering that emptying out glycogen is part of our natural design, allowing the food we then eat to be used or stored as fuel, and not get added to our waists.

When glycogen stores are full, eating too much will rapidly make you fatter. Training to failure is draining, and although direct evidence doesn't exist, it's likely to make you feel *overtrained* if you hit failure non-stop. In a full-body workout, it's true that the earlier exercises slightly benefit from your highest energy levels. The drop-off in energy towards the end isn't nearly as bad as people claim, but going to failure on every set would be a push too far for most.

With all these benefits, and some drawbacks, it's smart to take a balanced approach. Here's what you need to do:

On the <u>last</u> set of each exercise, aim for failure. Do this if it's safe, and don't let your form get too loose.

The <u>goal</u> isn't to *chase* failure, it's to keep going until you hit a wall. There's a difference. We're not about *feeling the burn*. We are about *finding the limits*. Going to failure won't necessarily be all fireworks and screaming "yeah buddy, light weight". Sometimes it's a quiet thing - a <u>sudden</u> stop - that no one else around you will even notice. I'll say it again:

Hitting failure isn't about screaming, or feeling the burn. It's simply about being unable to get another good rep.

And here's something that needs its own line:

Hitting failure takes honesty.

You must be *honest* and ask the question, can I get another rep? If the answer is *yes*, and if you're feeling in control, go for it.

It will boost growth. And, this one last set to failure will help you accurately know your true strength levels, because when your numbers go up on *that* set, the improvement becomes instantly memorable.

BRO VS PRO

bro

✗   training to failure is old school and unnecessary
✗   training to failure is dangerous
✗   training to failure is only good if you do it all the time

pro

✓   training to failure on your last set boosts muscle growth
✓   training to failure helps control body fat and improve health
✓   training to failure takes concentration and honesty

BUILDING YOUR REP

One of the commonest training mistakes is getting poor *quality* reps. In a bodybuilder's world, the rep is like the atom, i.e. the smallest part of their workout. And it's the most crucial. **You are only as good as your rep**. You can go high or low volume, full-body or splits, train 6 days or just Mondays, but *none* of it matters unless you master *the rep*.

The *perfect rep* is made up of two halves:

- correct speed
- mind-muscle connection

Let's deal with the need for speed, i.e. correct amount of it. If a muscle is getting shorter, it's called a **concentric contraction**. If it's getting longer, it's an **eccentric contraction**. If you are *holding* a weight anywhere in the rep, it's an **isometric contraction**. All of these are important.

CONCENTRIC CONTRACTION

In a dumbbell curl, it's where you curl it up. If you do this too fast, you'll probably use too much swing. At the same time, you'll work your lower back muscles, and if you're really bad, your front delts (shoulders). You will waste the opportunity to squeeze blood *through* the muscle, something which itself causes growth. Scientists call this **sarcoplasmic hypertrophy.** Hypertrophy means *growth*, and the sarcoplasm is the area of fluid in and around a muscle cell.

Boost this, and the muscle grows in size. There is some controversy in science about this, but undeniably, some muscle growth does happen without any change in strength.

A carefully controlled concentric contraction squeezes fluid through muscles and increases this kind of growth. Lift *too fast* and you probably aren't squeezing and getting maximum benefit. If you lift *too slowly*, there isn't much benefit either. The reps and set takes too long, you burn lots of internal carbs (glycogen), and you bubble up so much lactic acid that you ruin your technique. You reduce the overall amount of reps you get, which is bad for growth. With lactic acid levels high, you'll also damage the other half of the rep, namely...

ECCENTRIC CONTRACTION

Back to the dumbbell curl example, an eccentric contraction is where you're *lowering* the dumbbell. As a muscle lengthens, it gets slimmer, skinnier, *narrower*. And yet the weight is still the same. This same level of tension - *in a narrower space* - causes massive damage. And it's this damage that stimulates a different kind of growth. Scientists call it **myofibrillar hypertrophy**. Again, *hypertrophy* means growth, and the myofibril is just a tiny sliver of fiber which makes up muscle. They're like the threads string is made from. Make them bigger, and the whole muscle gets bigger. Make those bigger, and you'll need to get bigger t-shirts.

Myofibrillar hypertrophy is thought to last almost permanently. In steroid using athletes, much of the growth can be sarcoplasmic hypertrophy, and that seems to disappear easily. Two athletes at the same weight and measurements might *look* different due to their varying ratios of sarcoplasmic and myofibrillar hypertrophy. Those with myofibrillar hypertrophy look especially hard.

Back to the rep. If you lower a weight too fast, without control (or say, drop like a stone on a pull-up, i.e. where lats lengthening), you won't create *enough* damage.

Lowering the weight fast is a problem with most reps. Lower like you're the boss for maximum growth.

You should actively *feel* the muscle strain as you lower it. If you feel nothing, it's likely your muscle cells feel nothing either, and therefore there's no reason for them to grow.

Some of you might be wondering, why not just go *super* slow? A few years ago, this briefly became a popular training method. You could even see some doing it today, taking 30 seconds to do *one* rep. The problem with these is that they create massive muscle soreness. I'm not talking about a little stiffness, I mean, fall down the stairs kind of pain. This is not good, because you would have to reduce your overall **frequency** of working out. And it's vital that you do that, so that protein synthesis (growth) is happening for the majority of your time. If you're so sore you can't work out, you will spend too much time with Average Joe protein synthesis, i.e. you'll just maintain.

Also, less scientifically yet still important, is that an excessively long eccentric contraction means *less time on the lifting part*. And it's the concentric contraction, the *s-q-u-e-e-z-e*, that's most enjoyable. When research has been conducted into training either *fully* concentric or *fully* eccentric, it seems that instead, a balanced approach using both works well for most people.

Before we recommend a speed, what about the non-speedy bit of the rep?

ISOMETRIC CONTRACTION

On a dumbbell curl, the isometric part is anywhere you pause, but usually it's at the "top" of the rep. Your bicep won't change how long it is, but you're still sending an electrical impulse to it, keeping the blood pumped up, and stopping the dumbbell from making its descent.

It's a crucial and underrated part of every rep. Most trainees simply don't contract their muscles hard enough. Science hasn't found much evidence to show that an isometric contraction causes muscle growth, but it's still important. Why?

The isometric part of your rep - the squeeze and hold - builds *mind-muscle* connection. Along with lifting at the correct speed, this is the other half of a perfect rep.

If you consistently always pause your rep and squeeze at the end of the movement, you'll quickly build a strong mind-muscle connection. This link between our brains and muscles gets stronger the harder you work it. Done well, you'll develop an *immensely* muscular body, as you'll be able to target muscles like a sniper.

If you take an exercise like the dumbbell row, 99% of trainees feel their biceps and grip, and *some* of their lats. Those in the 1% feel their lats pumped and *hardly* feel their arms at all. That's how the dumbbell row is supposed to feel. It's no coincidence that on complex back and leg movements, people go through the motions and struggle to build a strong mind-muscle connection. These body parts are weak compared to most guys' chests and arms, areas where a strong isometric *squeeze* seems easy.

If you - pause - at the peak of every exercise, i.e. where the muscle is *shortest*, you'll increase your strength *fast*. This itself allow more reps, more damage, more stimulation, and quick growth. The harder your contraction, the more the body sends electrical signals to that muscle. Eventually, harder contractions give you more "electrical cables" at the ends of your muscle, which then enable even more fine-tuned control and power. Sport science calls this *motor end plate proliferation*. I call it a reward for training honestly. Also, pausing for a solid squeeze makes it *much* easier to feel the eccentric (lengthening) part of your rep.

Many new trainees hear the word *isometric* and think of the old time strongmen, especially one called *Charles Atlas*. He sold a strength training course based just on isometrics, calling it *Dynamic Tension*. It had a famous comic strip advertisement where a "97 pound weakling" builds up his body, and gets revenge on the bully who kicked sand in his face. Considering Mr Atlas based an *entire* training course on this part of the rep, it's a shame that few modern guys take the isometric part seriously.

Let's state it clearly:

All parts of the muscle contraction are important.

THE GOLDILOCKS SPEED

So how fast or slow should your reps be? The answer is in the nursery rhyme about *Goldilocks* and her ideal porridge. Don't remember? It's not too hot, not too cold, but *just* right. Translated into *Super Swole* language, it means:

The perfect rep speed is: <u>moderate</u>. 2 seconds up, a <u>definite pause</u> to show the weight who's the boss, and 2 seconds down.

If you go much faster or slower than this, it gets dangerous, boring, unproductive, *or all three.*

The one exception is your final set and rep.

THE FINAL COUNTDOWN

Your final set of each exercise will hopefully be taken to *positive failure*, i.e. where you can't push or pull any more. For most of this set, still use the *Goldilocks* speed. That's a couple of seconds to contract the muscle (lift) - a <u>pause</u> - and then a couple of seconds to lengthen it (lower). But on the *last few reps*, and definitely on the last one, **push as fast as you can**. In reality, because the weight is heavy, you *won't* move it fast. In fact, you'll be moving it slowly. But squeezing hard as you can, and *aiming* for fast, causes your fastest of fast twitch muscle fibers to fire.

Push fast on your last reps. It won't move fast, but it will activate the most powerful muscle fibers you own.

After this, don't waste the final eccentric part of your final rep. For example, if you're holding dumbbells, don't just let them drop like stones onto the floor. Or if you're on a pull-up, don't just jump off the bar once you've touched your nose to it. Be cool, be the boss of the movement, and lower slowly. I'm not secretly steering you away from injury by the way. I'm keen for you to not miss out on growth. The *last-half of the last-rep* builds mind-muscle connection, confidence, and growth. Wimping out isn't honest. Remember, be the boss.

GET A GRIP

If you're finding all this theory talk difficult to apply, here's a tip. Before you start each exercise, i.e. before your first rep, *get a grip*. I mean, **make a ritual out of finding the perfect hand or foot placement on the bar or machine**. Try to use the same bars and machines if possible, for consistency.

But even if you're forced to use something else, make a point of having a <u>pre-rep ritual</u>. Watch most guys, and you'll notice that once they feel ready for the next set, they simply jump to it like chimps playing in a zoo.

Your mind-muscle connection is massively enhanced if you take a moment, and develop a ritual to find the perfect position. Once you find it - *lock it down* - and begin.

After a few workouts this becomes a great habit, and you'll be surprised about how much extra strength it gives you. So next time you do your lat pulldowns, don't just jump on like a chimp. Find your spot, wrap the fingers of one hand *precisely* around it, do the other hand carefully too, and **bang**, you're set. Try it and see. You'll be a beast, and never go back.

BRO VS PRO

bro

- ✗ rep speed doesn't matter
- ✗ the lifting / lowering is the most important part
- ✗ isometrics are for old-time strongmen

pro

- ✓ using the optimal rep speed is crucial for growth
- ✓ eccentric and concentric contractions affect muscle differently
- ✓ isometric contractions build a strong mind-muscle connection

TAKING ORDERS

How you order your exercises may feel important. You can do it how you like, and it probably wouldn't make *much* difference long-term, but there are some guidelines.

TRAIN LEGS LAST (ALMOST)

A full-body workout is a tough workout, a man's workout (a tough woman's too). Most of your non-leg exercises actually require your legs to stay strong as a base. Even dumbbell curls suffer if your legs are shaky.

So although it seems unusual, there's definite logic in training legs *last*. Of course, legs are known for being a tough body part to train, and this is actually a good reason to put them last. Although you'll be tired compared to the freshness found at the beginning, training them last means you can give them your all, and not worry about being wiped out for the remaining 90% of your workout.

If you are including squats of some kind, they literally should be your last exercise. Squats are designed to challenge your quads, hams and glutes, but even the best squatter in the world *can't* stop their lower and middle spine from being worked. It's your body's hinge, and if you exhaust it before your other exercises, everything suffers. Squat last. Well, almost.

ABSOLUTELY LAST

I would put abs after legs. Why?

Because they affect your ability to keep your middle tight during large leg movements like squats. Keeping tight during leg movements is important for safety. Having an exhausted core before you squat will reduce overall effort. It can also reduce your performance on exercises like one-arm rows, floor press, press (shoulder presses) and yet again, dumbbell curls (these little guys really are sensitive). By the way, if you can manage hanging leg-raises as your last exercise, they'll help decompress your spine, which may have become compressed (squashed down) during squats.

As abs are postural muscles (i.e. they help you keep a normal posture), and made for endurance, they don't need or like a heavy weight. This means you'll easily be able to perform ab movements before you hit the changing rooms. Some exercises like hanging leg-raises, also involve the hip flexors. These are muscles are the opposite of those used in the squat (hip extensors). This nicely rounds out a routine.

PUT SMALLER BODY PARTS AFTER MAJOR

For a while, it was trendy to train biceps *before* back. The theory was that by the time you did your pulldowns or rows, your tired biceps wouldn't be able to help, and therefore you'd feel it in your lats more. Research eventually showed this was a bad idea, with back muscle growth actually suffering long-term. I'll add this if you can't feel your back muscles, it's time to re-think your technique.

So whenever possible, train smaller parts like biceps, triceps, shoulders and abs, *after* your chest and back. This also suits the program, because by the time you hit the smaller muscles, they're partially trained.

Apart from these guidelines, it's fine to shift things around as you wish. There might be times when the gym is busy and you can't hit the order you like. Just roll with it.

And there will be other times when you *want* to play with things, perhaps because you sense one muscle needs a bit more priority. Use your common sense, and have fun too.

BRO VS PRO

bro

- ✗ kill your small muscles first so the bigger ones feel more later
- ✗ train legs first because they need more energy
- ✗ always stick to an exact order of exercises

pro

- ✓ train legs last so you don't ruin 90% of your workout
- ✓ train chest and back before triceps, biceps and shoulders
- ✓ training out of your normal order won't kill you

RISE OF THE MACHINES

Ask someone who works out, "are free weights better than machines?" and 99% of them will say "yes". Must be true, right? Nope. It's what they were told by their gym seniors, and so, they simply re-tell that to others. To be fair, gyms often divide themselves with small guys on the machines and bigger guys in the middle of heavy iron. But this isn't proof of free-weight superiority. All bodies sense load, or what most people call *weight*. There are many ways to apply it, and none is naturally better than the other. **This section is important, especially before you go on to pick your actual exercises**. There's no point in discriminating against certain moves just because *broscience* says so.

FREE ADVICE

Some free weight exercises are brilliant, while others are awful. Take a barbell bench press. It's great, a solid exercise. Let's now consider the dumbbell flye. In theory, it's also good, as it does exactly what your pecs are designed for (horizontal adduction at the shoulder, aka: bringing your arm across your chest).

But in fact it only works the lower ranges, and is next to useless in every other portion. By the time your arms get a few inches above chest level, there's no fight against gravity, no damage, and therefore not much growth. It creates a pump due to the bottom-end stretch, but remember you need mechanical damage to stimulate growth fully. Because there's only resistance in the bottom range, you also develop a weakness in the rest of it, making dumbbell flyes unsatisfying overall.

THE CABLE GUY

Cables provide options that simply couldn't exist before them. Take a mid-height (chest height) *cable cross*. Free weights cannot recreate it, and no other movement provides the same level of resistance *throughout* the entire range of motion. No matter where your hand is, the weighted stack is being lifted directly against gravity, creating damage (future growth). This is basically a standing up dumbbell flye, but with cables. It turns a so-called isolation exercise into an outstanding muscle builder.

Cables also allow you to work around an injury. A painful lower back makes it difficult to pick up dumbbells or a barbell and get into position. Because the weight using cables is the stack, all you need to do is select your weight with the pin and get into a good position *before* you take on any load. This small but crucial difference saves you if you're injured.

THE GOOD, THE BAD, AND THE UGLY

Modern machines can go from very bad to very good. *Hammer Strength* for example, make many pieces that perfectly blend free weight and machine. And yet even with that company, some of their machines could feel uncomfortable. If you're lucky, a particular brand or machine might fit you perfectly.

There may be a time when it helps to use a machine the *wrong* way around, or off to one side slightly. Doing this could get you strange looks, or it might even get you in trouble with the gym management. Who cares, as long as it produces gains. Some machines are actually dangerous the "right" way around. And some go from being dangerous or average the right way around, to being brilliant the "wrong" way around. Some bi-lateral machines (i.e. machines with two moving handles for your left *and* right arms / legs) become great uni-lateral machines.

By taking a *decent* two-handed machine row for example, and using it one-handed, you can fine-tune your body's positioning and make it a *brilliant* exercise. Don't always be limited by a machine's instructions or how others use it.

Some machines allow you to progress onto free weights with more safety, and much more mind-muscle connection. If for example you can't dip your body weight, a dip machine will help you get there. The same can be said for lat pulldowns helping your journey to bodyweight pull-ups. While you're using these assisted machines, you can really nail the mind-muscle connection. When you eventually do the *full* version, you will have superior *feel*, especially compared to guys who start with the heavy stuff and fail to feel the "targets". Never let your ego or fear of embarrassment get in the way of mastering an exercise.

ISOLATION DISCRIMINATION

While we're on the subject of machines, free weights and cables, it seems right to talk about *isolation vs compound* movements. An **isolation** exercise is easy to understand. It's where you generally hit one muscle. A dumbbell curl is often used as an example. In reality, no movement is a true isolation movement. The dumbbell curl hits the bicep, the brachialis (a big muscle underneath the bicep), the brachioradialis (the largest muscle of the forearm), and unless you're supported when doing it, it contracts your spinal muscles. It's not just a slight working of the lower back by the way, it's a lot. Without your lower back contracting hard, it would literally be impossible to hold even a 20 pound dumbbell in the mid position. Science rant over, let's assume isolation means *isolation*.

And then there's the big daddy, **compound**. This means using multiple muscles and multiple joints. Bench press, pulldown and the squat are all compound movements.

Now there's nothing wrong with compound movements in general, just like there's nothing wrong with isolation movements, in general. The problem arises when we treat them like royalty, and assume they can do no wrong. For those who live in England, it's obvious that the royalty can do wrong!

We tend to assume all compound exercises as being extremely productive, natural, safe, and good for beginners. They can be productive, and sometimes they mimic natural movements. But just because cavemen did something similar *doesn't* mean we have to. Cavemen also ate the brains of other humans! Getting swole is unnatural in some ways, so bringing out the "natural" love for compound movements is silly. They tend to be safer for certain muscles than some isolation movements - but overall - they can also be dangerous.

And that also means their "good for beginners" tag is inaccurate. The so-called basics, compound movements like squats and bench press, take years to perfect. As well as hyping up compounds, broscientists tend to mock isolation movements. This is also a silly stance to take. Because:

If you hit a muscle hard, with good mind-muscle connection and a bit of metabolic stress, it will be stimulated to grow.

That - is - *it*. Compounds can save you time in the gym, and burn more calories per breath of effort, but so what. Some isolation movements are undeniably good. They're snipers that hit the targets machine guns can miss. You will get some bicep growth from pull-ups or pull-downs (even though you should really feel lats), but they can never work like a good curl. And although your abs work during a push-up, the specialized treatment of a hanging leg-raise is unbeatable.

LOAD OF RUBBISH

Finally, it's worth adding that although weight is important to create good damage, it's not just about the numbers. Your body is a system of levers (and so are some machines). A military press can involve some pretty hefty poundages compared to a dumbbell side raise. This often causes guys to say "you can use more weight with the press, so it's better for your delts". Well, you can use more weight because you're using the shoulders *and* the triceps *and* the chest *and* possibly your legs. You use less on a side raise because it's *just* shoulders. You also struggle with a "light" weight because the load is at the end of a long lever (your arm). In that mechanically poor position, your 15-pound dumbbell becomes good at creating damage. Your arm in the military press will be bent at the elbow, making the lever mechanically good, and hence it's much easier to move the weight. You see: **it's not weight in itself, but the relative stress on the muscle.**

If you want a simple explanation using machines, consider this. You can load up a leg press with 300 pounds, and many guys will be able to move it. But stick 300 on a barbell, and hardly any can squat down. Why? Because the design of a leg press machine, being at a slope, takes lots of the weight off (anywhere from you actually moving 70% to just 30% of the weight!). That doesn't make the leg press bad and the squat good. It means you need slightly more weight on the leg press to feel the same pressure in your quads as you'd get on the squat. It means you need a 15-pound dumbbell to fry your delts in a side raise compared to say 60 pounds needed if using a military press.

Weight is weight, and gravity is gravity, but different factors like the design of a machine, your body's position against gravity, and your body's leverage, all affect what your body *feels* in terms of load.

Although you should always strive to increase the weights you're using over time, the number itself isn't critical; <u>it's how hard your muscle is working</u> (i.e. the harder the better).

That sentence should stop you worrying about compound movements vs. isolation, free weights vs. machines, and the total weight being lifted. **It's all about the *application* of weight.** Make mind-muscle connection your best friend.

The point of this section isn't just to chitchat about the obvious. It's to ram home the message that there's a tool for every job. And that *no* particular tool is good or bad. It's either right for that job, or not right for that job. Don't let anyone convince you otherwise. Let's sum up:

Don't discriminate between types of equipment or how one exercise is more "macho" than another. Experiment to find the best tool for the job - <u>work it hard</u> - and strive to build up the weight bit by bit.

BRO VS PRO

bro

- ×   machines are bad/good
- ×   free weights are the only way to build mass seriously
- ×   cables are for girls

pro

- ✓   machines & free weights are good/bad depending on the job
- ✓   weight on the bar/stack isn't proof of a muscle working hard
- ✓   cables allow you to explore unique exercise possibilities

THE SWOLE ROUTINE

You've waded through nine chapters so far, and are probably desperate to put something together. So, here's the final piece of the puzzle for now. Be sure to read beyond this section though, as there's lots of stuff on diet and more. To put a routine together, **pick <u>one</u> exercise from <u>each</u> of these sections**.

CHEST

Flat dumbbell bench press
Flat barbell bench press
Flat chest press (plate-loaded/weight stack)
Dip (bodyweight/machine/plate-loaded/supported)
Mid-height standing cable flye

BACK

Lat pulldown to front (wide overhand/parallel/plate-loaded)
Pull-up (wide overhand/parallel/supported)
Seated row (cable/plate-loaded/machine)
One-arm dumbbell row (standing supported/bench)
T-bar row (supported)

THIGHS

Trap/Shrug bar squat
Barbell squat
Leg Press (plate-loaded/weight stack)
Hack squat
Dumbbell squat (regular/goblet/hip belt)

SHOULDERS

Military Press
Dumbbell shoulder press (alternate/two-handed/one-handed)
Cable side-raise
Dumbbell upright row (one-handed)
Machine press (plate-loaded/weight stack)

BICEPS

Barbell curl
Dumbbell curl (alternate/two-handed/one-handed)
Hammer curl (alternate/two-handed/one-handed/Khanna curl)

TRICEPS

Cable pushdown (two-handed/one-handed/rope/V-bar)
Dumbbell lying tricep extension
Barbell lying tricep extension (EZ curl bar)

ABDOMINALS

Hanging leg raise
Swiss / stability ball crunch

SPINE

Back extension (bench)
Standing back roll (barbell/dumbbell)

You should now have:

• 3 major exercises (chest, back, thighs)
• 3 minor exercises (biceps, triceps, shoulders)
• 2 core exercises (one for abs, one for spine)

Done that? You're ready to go! Hold up, I said there's more stuff to read, so keep going. In the meantime, here's an example of what a routine could look like:

Dumbbell bench press	*6 x 4-10*
Lat pulldowns to the front	*6 x 4-10*
Military press	*3 x 4-10*
Hammer curl	*3 x 4-10*
Rope tricep pushdown	*3 x 4-10*
Leg press	*6 x 4-10*
Hanging leg raise	*2 x max (1st set is a 5 rep warm-up)*
Back extension	*1 x max (the spine will be warmed-up)*
Total sets	*30*
Total time	*1½ to 2 hours*
Total frequency	*Every third day to every other day*
	(10 to 15 times per month)

Remember, **this is *just* an example**. A great routine is one you enjoy. Start by picking *exercises* you enjoy, one for each major muscle group. You may find that some of your favorites don't get on with other favorites. Experiment, play. Once you find the moves you like, get into the gym and work them hard.

PERFECT FORM

Although a book can't beat careful experience in the gym, it can give you a few pointers. You'd think that with all the forums and *YouTube*, everyone would have amazing technique. But they don't.

On average, for every 20 guys you see, only 1 will have *flawless technique*. Surprisingly, only a few have really *dangerous* technique. But where does that leave the rest? Well, most people are just so-so technique wise. And that's what their bodies look like: so-so. Meh! Even if you take drugs and grow from poor technique, using great technique will get you there *much* faster. The goals of all good technique are simple:

Mind-muscle connection

and

Mind-muscle connection

It's not a typo, and I haven't forgotten about safety. You see, if you seek good mind-muscle connection, you will be safe. When *your* body gets used in its strongest positions and lines, you get a hard contraction, and you'll be safe. The word "your" is in italics because while good technique is good technique, there are slight variations due to the length of bones, where muscles attach, and how long your muscle fibers are. Some bodies are especially tight, and no matter how many sports therapists they pay, they'll always be that way. Some are the opposite. So it's up to you to *finesse* your exercise technique. Find subtle shifts in body, hand or foot position, and make it yours. **Own the exercise, be the boss.**

To get you on the right track, here are some thoughts on our key *Super Swole* exercise choices. By the way, they're not entire descriptions of the exercises - start to finish - but pointers on the parts most people get wrong.

CHEST

Flat dumbbell bench press

This is an excellent natural movement when performed correctly. The best way to get into position is to pick up the dumbbells, let them hang at your sides, and as you sit down, swing them slightly onto each mid-thigh area. When you're ready to press, kick up one knee then the other, and gradually get flat. If you find it difficult, it's usually possible to get one dumbbell into position and have someone pass you the other.

If you feel like you need a spot, you must find someone experienced. The dumbbell bench press needs the slightest of touches underneath your triceps. Because both arms move independent of each other, your spotter must be smart enough - *in real time* - to notice which side needs help. The safest way to put the dumbbells down is to drop them one side then the other.

Key pointers are that you press in a natural line, with elbows never too low or too high. Never force your arms away from your natural groove. With time, your natural groove will find its best path. Powerlifters encourage a low path, while some bodybuilders suggest bringing the elbows almost as high as your ear level. Avoid both extremes.

Push the dumbbells mainly straight up. That is, do not attempt to make them touch together in the middle. Do not let them sway out to the side either.

A natural groove is always straight up, with *slight* travel inwards (a few inches at most).

Also, avoid an excess stretch at the bottom. You may find that you naturally stop *before* chest level. If this feels enough of a stretch, it probably is. If going deeper feels too, consider using a *dumbbell floor press*. This is the same movement, just done on the floor. The floor prevents an excess stretch of the shoulders, and actually makes the best "bench" in the world. You'll be very stable, and very able to push hard. Just do it somewhere safe, i.e. inside the area of a Smith machine or power rack. This should prevent people dropping things on your face.

Flat barbell bench press

Much of the same advice for dumbbell bench applies here. It's a much easier exercise to get into, as you only need to de-rack the bar or have someone else hand it to you. Although it's easier to spot than dumbbell bench press, be sure to seek out an experienced person if you want one. I often see incorrect spotting that ranges from distracting chatter on every rep ("it's all you bro"), to where a spotter is actually lifting the bar so much, they're getting a shoulder workout.

Again, find a natural path with the barbell. Don't listen to those who say you should either "lower it to nipple level" or "press it to your neck". Find a natural line; it takes time. The path of the bar is not straight up and down. It tends to move slightly forward and then backwards as it's almost locked out. Again, don't look to create this, but don't be shocked when it happens. Try to be consistent by using the same bar regularly, and making a note of where your grip goes. Incidentally, with regards grip width, moderate is usually optimal. Too narrow hits the triceps, too wide hits (hurts) your shoulders. The strongest position will usually be the most biomechanically perfect. This is true of most muscles and their movements.

Flat chest press (plate-loaded / weight stack)

Of course machines vary, but the first advice is to find a nice hand position. With regards the seat, make sure you're at a level where pushing feels straight out in front of you, instead of your pecs being ultra tight (seat too low) or the contraction only being felt at the end (seat too high). Make a mental note of the position you find best, and generally stick to it, varying it only slightly by a notch from time to time.

With regards to hand placement, the main consideration is that at full stretch, you *aren't* too stretched. You don't want to feel too narrow and bunched up either. Like all machines, if you find it uncomfortable, go elsewhere. And if your gym is limited to that machine, consider using it one-handed. This way you can move your body *around it* slightly, and find a good line.

Dip (body weight / machine / plate-loaded / supported)

To use the dip for chest, you need slightly wide dipping bars. Ideally, V-shaped bars, wider at the end where you put your hands. A supported machine is great for learning technique. Don't let your arms bend so much that your lower and upper arm angle gets less than 90 degrees. If you're feeling "bunched" up at the bottom of a dip, you've gone too far. Overstretching the chest isn't necessary. It puts your shoulder area at risk.

Wrapping your thumbs over the bars helps improve mind-muscle connection in this movement. The strongest contraction occurs when your arms get closer to locking out. So, don't rush it. Always focus on the chest. The triceps get happy no matter what you do. Chest, chest, chest.

Mid-height standing cable flye

Sorry guys, but to do this you need a cable crossover unit that allows changes in the cable height. If you use the high handles of a regular cable crossover, you turn it into a kind of dip. And because of where the weight is pulling your arms, the rotator cuff muscles around your shoulders will strain slightly, potentially leading to an injury.

The ideal way to do this is one-handed, especially to learn the movement. Set the cable to match where you'd naturally put your arm out in front of you. If you can, use a rope handle, nylon loop, or even the cable's rubber stopper. Position yourself so that you pull no more than straight out to the side. An overstretched starting position is bad for shoulders and strength. It's better if your arm is slightly forward of being out to the side, i.e. slightly less stretched than where a dumbbell flye starts from.

Work through the movement smoothly and do not worry about crossing your arm completely over the chest's mid line. It's not necessary. Keep your arm fairly straight, and allow slightly more bend in the elbow on your heaviest set. The optimal groove is ever-so-slightly travelling downwards.

BACK

Lat pulldown to front (wide overhand / parallel / V bar / plate-loaded)

The traditional lat pulldown is a very effective exercise. It takes a classic movement, the pull-up, and makes it accessible for all. Set up the machine so that the seat is low enough to guarantee a good stretch. It is best to start by standing anyway, as it allows you to spend time on mastering your hand placement.

A moderately wide grip on a straight bar is usually best. Parallel or V-bars, also excellent, obviously dictate your grip width due to their handles. Back to the straight bar; consider using a thumbless grip. This is where you wrap your thumbs over the bar, with the intention of improving mind-muscle connection. When your hands are like "hooks", you tend to pull less with your biceps, and more with your lats. And remember, the pulldown is primarily for your back, not your arms.

Sit down with the bar, and feel the tension for a moment. Then lean back, somewhere between 30 and 45 degrees. Unless you have access to a mirror (or a friend who can tell you), this will simply "feel" like leaning back. When you feel slightly awkward, it's enough. Studies show that being slightly backwards increases the amount of your lats you hit. Pull smoothly, and aim to touch the bar to your *nose or chin*. Do not aim for the chest. That range of motion isn't necessary and tends to contract the biceps more near the end. Plus, it may rotate your arms forwards. Check out beginners to see extremes of this. They almost look like they're doing a wide-grip tricep pushdown. Avoid this at all cost. As said, just pull to the nose or chin.

When you release the bar, go *almost* all the way up. That is, don't let your arms fully lock out. Going that far tends to break the already fragile mind-muscle connection of the lats. Keep hitting them in this juicy mid-range, and they will grow fast. They'll get strong quick too.

If you opt for the V-bar or parallel bar attachment, still lean back, and aim to pull to slightly lower than your chin. You can even *aim* to hit your chest, although your flexibility may mean you don't actually touch it.

These bar attachments tend to shift the emphasis of where you hit the lats (from upper and lower areas, to middle). Don't change handles from workout to workout. Use one for at least 6 weeks before switching (unless an injury forces a change earlier).

Pull-up (wide overhand / parallel / V bar / supported)

The pull-up's main advantage over the lat pulldown, is the extra increase in eccentric loading (your muscles lengthening under a weight). If you are using anything other than the supported version, you need to find a way of getting into position carefully. I am not talking about avoiding injury. It's about being able to set yourself up on the bar properly. You need to get an excellent grip to enhance your mind-muscle connection. If you have to *jump* to get the bar, the beginning of the set will feel rushed, and you won't have the same level of focus compared to setting yourself up carefully. Find a way (e.g. a step, nearby ledge or even friend). Once in position, consider using a thumbless grip. On "pulling" movements, it's safe. Avoid a thumbless grip on anything else though.

Try to start the pull with your lats. To do this, it helps to not overstretch at the bottom of the movement. Your biceps, forearm muscle (brachioradialis) and under-the-bicep muscle (brachialis) are too weak to help in this position, and the lats are out of position also. Only a small muscle (teres major) can work. You're better off doing pull-ups with what looks like a poor technique: i.e. only going to about 80% of the normal bottom position. This way you can pull with the lats more, and contract them harder as you rise. The biceps will always help (and so will the pecs and triceps to some degree), but at least the lats will be in a strong line to pull. When you do pull, you do *not* have to clear your chin over the bar. Pulling to the nose is fine, and in most cases, best. It's the middle range of pull-ups that hits the "belly" of the main muscles.

Seated row (cable / plate-loaded / machine)

All variations of this exercise should start the same way. Grab the handles or attachment, and then rock back to sit down.

By the time you sit, there should be tension on your lats. If you are on a cable row, pull the handle fairly low. Your guideline is not really where your arms are, but where you feel you hit *most* of the lats. If you're on a plate-loaded seated row, or other machine, you'll have to adjust the seat height and possibly your hand position to get it right. All seated rows hit the lats, as well as the middle of your trapezius, and rhomboid muscles. Rows, i.e. horizontal pulling (as opposed to pulldowns and pull-ups which are vertical pulls), hit more of the "back" as a whole.

Do not be tempted to lean very far forward, even if you did see Arnold do it in *Pumping Iron*. Doing this creates a truly all round "back" exercise, but for your spine to survive it you really need to know what you're doing. Let the spine get worked in other ways, and focus on lats. A slight forward lean gives them some useful stretch (like leaning back in the pulldown), but that's about it.

One-arm dumbbell row (standing supported / bench)

In theory, a simple exercise. In reality, it's not. Most people look like they're starting a speedboat's engine when doing it. If instead you want your lats to grow full throttle, listen up. To make your lats contract, you have to pay special attention to the *beginning* of the movement. Get that right, and the exercise takes care of itself. When *starting* the pull, think about your lats doing it. Willingly try to *not* use your biceps. The lat muscles attach to your upper arm bone, and if you can send the nerve impulse to them, it will start the movement. If this all sounds complicated, remember this: your bicep muscle should not feel like it's getting much shorter during a row. The lower part of your arm should almost feel as if it's just hanging loosely, with all the movement coming from the shoulder joint. If you find your arms tired on rows, you are doing it wrong. At most, they can help assist in the final range of motion.

The dumbbell moves naturally back in an arc, from hanging out in front of you, to being pulled towards your hips, knee or back leg. Once you pull, keep going, but you don't have to pull your elbow *behind* your back. Anyone watching you do it correctly might say your range of motion is too small. Ignore them. A long range of motion on rows is likely to reduce your mind-muscle connection in a flash. Keep your lats on fire.

If the elbow does travel behind the back level, it's your rear delts that power it. Plus, your bicep and forearm flexors. You don't want any of these muscles coming to the party. Keep a certain "looseness", locked on to the lat mind-muscle connection.

T-bar row (supported)

Originally, the T-bar row was always unsupported. Thankfully, most gyms fear of health and safety problems moved towards the chest-supported version. The unsupported one, like the barbell row, is effective, but few trainees have the spinal and mental strength to do it justice.

Technique on the supported T-bar is fairly restricted by the machine itself, but it's still worth pointing out that the mind-muscle connection is decided by you. Start the movement by thinking about your lats pulling, not your biceps. If you feel biceps, you're either not concentrating hard enough, or you are trying too hard with an excessively long range of motion. This contraction too near the top forces your arms to take over.

If you find your breathing constricted to the point of distraction, consider another movement. I wouldn't want you to suffer and get into the habit of "peeling" away from the machine's chest pad just to breathe. We're not training lungs!

THIGHS

Trap / Shrug bar squat

The bar required for this type of squat is a smart invention. It takes the best parts of squats and deadlifts, and eliminates their weaknesses.

That is, it's a free weight exercise directly in line against gravity. It reproduces a natural movement, picking stuff up and squeezing with the legs, and yet it avoids the excess forward lean of some squats, and also misses the awkward hand position and lean of the deadlift. In short, it's a pure and as beastly a movement as you can get.

In fact, it's almost impossible to go wrong, technique wise. Due to the parallel handles and centering of body position, even a beginner can work hard on it. If you have poor ankle flexibility, instead of putting plates under your heels, try a shorter range of motion, and gradually increase it with time. Keep your head level, and try to push with a nice balance of muscle groups, i.e. push with glutes, hams and quads equally, while paying attention to keeping your back arched (contracted).

Use a mirror if possible, for left-to-right balance awareness, and have no fear of sticking your butt out as you dip down. The only problem with the shrug / trap bar, is that you can eventually build up to weights that challenge your grip. Straps can help, but the frustration of wrapping is often a deal-breaker for some. The good news is reaching that point takes a while.

So if you can, find a gym with this kind of bar, and make it your number one thigh movement.

This is the big daddy, although with trap / shrug bar on the scene, it's more like the granddaddy. Unlike the trap / shrug bar, there is potential for poor technique. Entire articles and books have been written on the squat. In my experience, squatters are born, and not made. You *can* be made into a great squatter, but it takes time, and it takes dropping your ego at the gym door.

Lighter weights are initially required to master technique. If you're on *Super Swole*, you might want to hunt down leg presses or shrug / trap bar squats to get the mass coming ASAP. The best squatters tend to have a good bone structure (average limb length), and high body-intelligence. *Body-intelligence* is an awareness of how your body feels and works. Some people really are blessed with fantastic "feel", and others (most) struggle. This quality is rare, and seems to be regardless of all other factors (ethnicity, what generation you're born in, age, gender, economic background, and even family; i.e. if one person has it, it's still rare for a brother, sister, mother or father to have it too).

Whatever your gifts, everyone can become a better squatter. The obvious mistakes are *leaning too far forwards*, *going too deep*, and *going too shallow*. Leaning forward too much is usually due to a couple of things. Excess weight too soon (before your spine has got strong enough), and poor hip flexibility. This improves by *conscientious* squatting. A good mental awareness of making all the body parts "concertina" (fold) at the same time helps. Put simply, everything should move together, with hips and knees bending at a roughly equal rate. When one moves faster or slower than the other, problems happen.

Putting plates under your heels helps technique in an instant, but it's a poor long-term solution. Going too deep is a rare mistake, as most lack the flexibility to get there. Going too shallow is common. This is usually pure ego, and slapping on weight you can't handle.

Going to a few inches *above* parallel is perfectly fine, and safe for the knees. It is <u>not</u> necessary to go "ass to grass" for knee health. Knee health is affected by many other factors to start with (genes, bodyweight in general, your job).

High-rep squats are not advised, as concentration is difficult to maintain, often leading to the spine collapsing on each rep. Also, the cardiovascular effects reduce focus even more. To learn squats, it's smarter to work in lower rep ranges, at least initially. Placing the bar too high or too low on your back creates other problems, so find a natural placement, and stick to it. Finally, don't get flash: use those collars!

Leg Press (plate-loaded / weight stack)

Leg press machines vary, so this can never be a comprehensive answer. The key point is **foot placement**. You never want them too high, too low, too narrow or too wide. *Too high* increases hamstring activation, and reduce the use of your quads. It also can cause a rocking of your pelvis, which may damage the spine. Because the weight isn't on top of your spine (like in a squat), you may not feel the damage happen *as* it happens. *Too low* foot placement isn't ideal either. You'll get more quad action, especially from the part that extends the leg at the end range of motion (the *vastus medialis* muscle, aka: "teardrop"). Ideally you want to feel that your *whole leg*, including glutes, is making the push happen. When you spread the load like that, the gains are quicker, and the injury risk, lower. *Too narrow* legs is damaging for the hips as your leg bones will be moving in diagonally inward path lines, and *too wide* placement will heavily tax your adductor muscles. There's nothing wrong with working leg adductor muscles in general, but they need to be balanced with leg abductor muscles too. Any time you imbalance opposing muscles, your body eventually will shut down progress in both to prevent further injury.

Do not allow your knees to come right into your chest. Doing this suggests you have bent your knees too far. Around a 90 degree angle between upper thigh and lower leg is fine. While the debate about squat depth and knee depth rages on, it's worth pointing out the obvious. I have rarely - if ever - seen people with injuries through using reduced ranges of motion, but I have seen *many* with injuries from an excessive range. If a joint has a great range of motion when unloaded, it doesn't mean it's meant to do the same with weight.

Leg presses often get loaded with tons of plates, which looks cool. Don't delude yourself, as due to physics, you're actually lifting between 70 and 30% of that! So, drop the ego off at the gym door, and focus on *smooth* reps with a strong mind-muscle connection.

Do not go for constant tension, i.e. non-stop reps, even if that feels addictive. Push a rep, pause at the top, lower slowly, micro pause with knees approaching the chest, *go again*. And please, when you're finished using all those plates, take them off. The leg press is designed to train your legs, not others' forearms and back!

Hack squat

Inspired by the 19th and 20th century Russian / German strongman *George Hackenschmidt*, this movement is like a squat, and also like a leg press, with you inside the machine. The German word *hacke* also means "heel".

Be warned: people find that the weight feels very different on hacks, compared to leg press, and even compared to regular barbell squats. They find it feels heavy! Again, the main consideration is foot placement. You don't want them too far up on the footplate, or you'll hit hams and glutes a bit too hard. If you have your feet too far under you, you'll hit quads hard, but you may also damage the patellar tendon of your knee.

In fact, for some reason, incorrect foot placement on hack squats is the number one problem with it. If you find a sweet spot, find a way of sticking to it.

Because balance is taken out of the equation, many trainees are tempted to bring their feet very close together. This is still not recommended. That position doesn't occur in nature. At the same time, an excessively wide stance over works your inner thighs (adductors).

Dumbbell squat (regular / goblet / hip-belt)

These are often seen as weak relations to the barbell, but they have a place, especially for variety, and even more so in those who might have an injury. The goblet squat and hip-belt squat allow for a safer placement of the weight. It goes through the center of the body, much like the trap / shrug bar.

This allows the back to be kept upright, and more of the load to hit the thighs. Hip-belt squats need little help regarding technique. They are slow to set up, but *very* natural once you're doing them.

Goblet squats also are straightforward. It's worth pointing out that in the traditional goblet squat, the weight will eventually get so heavy, that holding the dumbbell becomes tiring. If you then switch to the sumo-style goblet squat, i.e. holding a dumbbell at arms length, excess forward lean could creep in. You have to be honest with your technique in these movements, and it's unlikely any gym or staff member will correct you (they probably won't know what you're doing).

The dumbbell squat is incredibly natural. Even in poor barbell squatters, dumbbells tend to produce better technique, with excess forward lean or heels off the floor coming much later. Again, the problem with dumbbell squats is that they become a victim of their own success.

When the weight your legs and back can handle gets high enough, your forearms, hands, traps and side delts start complaining.

The logical place for dumbbell squat and their variants is early in a plan, especially to get your hips and knees moving in unison, i.e. together. Once you've got some heavy mileage out of them, accept that it's time to move to alternative movements.

SHOULDERS

Military Press

A classic movement that in today's "functional fitness" environment looks almost cartoon-like. It's simply a barbell shoulder press in front of you. Done correctly, it's effective at building delts, triceps, upper chest, and even abdominal wall strength.

There are few pointers, other than finding a strong base to push from, typically shoulder width spacing for your legs, and slightly wider than shoulder width for your arms on the bar. With the barbell *almost* resting at upper chest level, shoot for spacing whereby your forearms are roughly at right angles to the floor. Put simply, where your forearms are almost straight up (as opposed to pointing left or right).

Try to avoid an excessive backwards lean, simply because you will be on the edge of worrying about toppling backwards, and therefore having a poor mind-muscle connection in general. But, a *slight* backwards lean is more desirable than literally appearing military in terms of body stiffness. Lower the bar - carefully - to chin or almost upper chest level. An excessive range of motion will feel instinctively strange, with your elbows seeming "bunched up" into your sides or travelling backwards. Hold a pause at the top, softly locking out if you can.

If and when you can manage that lock out, the bar will drift backwards over your head. This is the bar's natural path. Don't panic.

The problem with the military press is that eventually, the weight needed may be too heavy to get into position. If you have access to a power rack, walk-in squat rack, or even specialized press bench, it won't be a problem. If not, you may have to switch exercises at some point. Huffing and puffing before you start pressing is energy wasting, and potentially dangerous to your back and shoulders (or even other gym members). Of course, there are ways to get the weight overhead using various Olympic lifting moves, but that's beyond the scope of this book. In a nutshell, enjoy military presses while you can.

Dumbbell shoulder press (alternate / two-handed / one-handed)

The dumbbell shoulder press performed correctly is a thing of beauty. Well, maybe not beauty, but seeing great form is as rare as nice scenery, especially in gym landscape. Getting dumbbells into position can be a problem, but slightly less so than the problems with military press. There are ways to kick or knee them up, and of course a spotter can hand you *one* fairly safely if you go seated.

Incidentally, seated presses, while strict, aren't necessarily safer for your spine. There is a tendency to relax and round the spine when seated, compared to the natural tendency to contract and arch it hard when standing. Although the standing version feels tiring, it is safer for the spine. It will also build more bone density, something useful for long-term health.

With dumbbells, the main advantage is that both arms (and hence shoulders and traps) work independently. That's obvious. The other advantage, is elbow position. With a barbell, you *must* have your elbows fairly far back, towards being in a straight line.

With dumbbells, you can bring them slightly forward, which is more natural. Now, you can also move your wrists. This may feel useful, and it might be, but the main safety and performance improvements come from the *elbow placement*. Pay attention to them on lighter sets, and you'll understand. Do not bring them too far forwards, or you will change the emphasis of the exercise to front delts, upper chest, and much more tricep. This isn't bad in itself, but these areas are worked well enough elsewhere.

One-armed presses are particularly useful for building a strong mind-muscle connection to the delt, an area some actually find difficult to feel with a press. If you go this route, you may find it's necessary to hold onto something with your non-working arm. Then again, you may be a balance star, and be cool just standing and pressing.

A great advantage of a one-sided press, is the massively increased uppermost range of motion. This does help contract the delts harder, but it particularly hits the traps too. This is because when you truly reach overhead, the traps contract to rotate your shoulder blades. With strong delts and strong traps, you are sure to look a beast at the pool. You'll be fully functional for a game of water volleyball too.

Cable side raise

If possible, use a height adjustable cable unit, and set the cables at hand level, i.e. where your hand is by your side when standing up. This way, there's tension on your shoulder muscles right from the start. It will feel like you've set it up way too low before you give it a go. This variation is rarely seen in gyms, but produces very strong shoulders.

If you only have low cable attachments, they can still work. For either set-up, a rope works better than the traditional stirrup handle. If not the rope, then you can grasp the end of the cable itself. It usually has a rubber stopper to grip around.

And remember, the weights on the stack won't be hugely challenging for your grip. Standing side-on to the machine, your palms (using the rope) will face forward. This externally rotated position is safest for your shoulders, and very productive. If you have a regular stirrup handle, your palms will face your thighs. Never face your palms backwards, or use the "pour water out of a jug" technique at the top of the movement. This is internal rotation, and potentially destructive to your whole shoulder.

If you have the regular low cable attachment, raise your almost-straight arms to when they naturally run out of range. This is likely to be higher than parallel to the ground. Most people tell you to stop at this point. Ignore them! The shoulder is designed for mobility, and under strict control it can take it. If you can make it to 45 degrees above parallel, go for it. It is safe. If you have set up a mid-level attachment (about knee height), you will only get to about parallel, and that's fine. You make up for the smaller range by having *lots* of tension at the start.

The side delt, which this hits, is a small area of muscle. And, your arm is a long lever. This means: don't worry about the weight looking light. It's actually heavy. If the stack's weights jump up too much, find a way of placing small weights on it, to reduce the jumps.

Done correctly, cable side raises will massively improve your shoulders, making them round, and giving your entire physique a powerful presence. Plain old dumbbell side raises are still good, but cables are *great* and deserve their place in the pantheon of shoulder movement classics.

Dumbbell upright row (one-handed)

The traditional barbell upright row is rarely seen in today's gyms. It is still seen in "body pump" type aerobic classes, but the loads are very light.

The movement got a bad rep for damaging shoulders, and also got outshined by "modern" exercises like side raises. In reality, the upright row in *dumbbell* form is a great exercise. In effect, it *is* a side raise, with very bent arms. It's a compound version of the side raise (using delts *with* arm flexors). And performed in a loose-but-controlled style, it's effective. By varying body position, that's leaning "away" or "forwards", you can shift the emphasis around the highly mobile shoulder area.

It is a difficult movement to explain in words, and even in the gym, other than saying it's a one-hand upright row. An excellent way to develop a feel for it, is to carry bags (grocery bags) around on a long enough walk. As you start to get tired shoulders, try a few loose reps. It sounds strange, but a key function of the side delts is to hold heavy loads out to the side *when we're moving*. So, instead of being embarrassed, imagine you're a true caveman walking down the street! Try leaning away from the bag, and almost casually lifting it up to shoulder level. You *want* to use a mix of arms and shoulders here. Even with the arms helping, this natural movement can absolutely fry the shoulders. If you don't fancy using a grocery bag, pick up a moderate dumbbell, and walk around the gym for a while.

Once the lactic acid starts to build up, stop walking, and give it a go. In time, you can do it straight away, with no weird walk necessary, and no lactic acid to guide you.

In terms of progression, this movement can be loaded heavily. You must find the right groove, but because you're *sharing* the weight with arm flexors, the total load can keep going up for quite a while. Sharing between arm flexors and delts also means you will be better able to tolerate the jumps in dumbbell weights.

Machine press (plate-loaded / weight stack)

Machines and shoulders seem like a bad mix.

The former are mechanical, and rigid, while the latter is the peak of Mother Nature's design, free and fluid. But, if you find the *right* machine, it can be a perfect alternative to dumbbell presses and the military press. You give up a bit of stability, and for that, gain the ability to push strong along the movement's most productive lines.

It is crucial that for shoulder training on a machine, you find the right position. This may mean using the machine the "wrong" way around. Countless brands of machines seem to be affected by this. In addition, you may find that an unusable machine becomes good by using *one side of it*, i.e. doing one-sided presses. This is mainly because you are not restricted by sitting or standing in the middle, and can instead move around to find the sweet-spot.

You may want to try a thumbless grip, which is normally *not* recommended for pressing movements. In the case of a machine, I will assume that losing your grip will not result in a danger. As I can't see what machine you're using, you will have to use your common sense. But a thumbless grip can increase mind-muscle connection and help target the delts ahead of triceps. Other than finding the right position, it's all about pumping out smooth reps.

Remember, you're using this to develop shoulders, not set records in the overhead press. The temptation with pressing is to load it up. Your priority should be to maximize gains in size, while retaining healthy shoulders.

BICEPS

Barbell curl (straight or EZ curl bar)

Find a natural width to grip the bar. It's likely to be around shoulder width, i.e. where your arms are at your sides.

A *wide* or *narrow* grip is generally best avoided. If your wrists hurt, consider trying the EZ curl bar. And if that still hurts, skip to dumbbells.

You don't have to curl right from the bottom. Starting with a slight bend in the arm isn't cheating. It's the optimal length for the bicep muscle. When the bicep works "in nature", it's never at full stretch. Curl until you feel the load lightens, and then mentally try to create a hard contraction. Avoid a backwards lean and jerk up. This doesn't injure backs as people think, as the weight's generally too light. But it will damage bicep growth, and potentially set up a long-term injury.

Dumbbell curl (alternate / two-handed / one-handed)

The legendary dumbbell curl exists for good reason: it still works, and it's enjoyable. There are endless technique pointers, but most of these become obvious by watching others in the gym. You will see all kinds of nonsense being dished out! The key thing is to curl with mind-muscle connection.

Too often it becomes a macho exercise, with everyone attempting to bang out PB-busting weights and reps. In reality, the biceps are small muscles, and need focus rather than beasting.

Cheating the weight is cheating your gains. An excessive swing means you're probably missing the bicep sweet-spot, which is quite small. You don't need full extension, that is, where your arm is completely locked straight. The bicep tendon has poor leverage in this position, and was never designed to pull from there. The biceps are designed to assist back muscles *once* a "pull" has been started and almost completed. To take advantage of this evolutionary design: stop just shy of full lockout. And in terms of the top end, you'll naturally reduce your effort when gravity no longer fights you. This slightly shorter range of motion is not cheating. It's sensible.

You may see guys with great arms, who appear to be cheating with a short range of motion on their curls. Drugs aside, it may be that they have good body intelligence and know how to target the sweet-spot.

Twisting the dumbbells, also known as supination, doesn't make much sense. Supination is a function of the biceps, but you'd need a dumbbell with uneven weight at one end to work this function. Otherwise you're simply spinning the dumbbell around a bit, and stressing your wrists.

If you are struggling to find a good mind-muscle connection, try seated curls, which increase strictness. Or go one-sided, and use your other hand to touch the bicep you're working. This tends to increase feel very quickly.

Hammer curl (alternate / two-handed / one-handed / Khanna curl)

The hammer curl, in all its flavors, is somehow the poor cousin of the regular palms up curl. In theory the *brachioradialis* (forearm) gets more stimulation, and the bicep gets less.

In reality - *especially after a few workouts* - most people find it's a hidden gem. In truth, it's hard to deny how natural the hammer position feels. In fact, most movements feel better in this "neutral" position. Without any tendency to twist the wrist, you just focus on lifting. It's important to get your grip in the center of the dumbbell, as being offset may eventually cause a strange wrist strain. Other than that, it's hard to go wrong with it.

An unusual but particularly good variation is the Khanna curl (named after British sport scientist Paul Khanna). This is a one-handed curl, where you place your non-working hand on a piece of equipment (e.g. barbell rack or exercise machine), somewhere around mid-torso height. This enables you to lean forwards slightly, hang the working arm loosely, and focus your attention on it nicely. It's a very natural and powerful position.

TRICEPS

Cable pushdown (two-handed / one-handed / rope / V-bar)

The twin or single rope is the best attachment for this exercise. Alternatively, there are nylon and fabric loops that also work well. The V-bar allows for heavy shifting of weight, but be careful, as it also encourages bad form. Stay away from straight bars, as they cannot accommodate the natural line of movement.

Find a position that's not very *close* to the stack, and not very *far* either. Close tends to make people go for a long range of motion, starting with their forearms bunched against their biceps. This overstretches the tricep tendon and will wreck your arms quicker than you can find a therapist. Also, standing too far away means stretching the tricep at its other end (it crosses the shoulder area).

While some stretching of a muscle is good, too much on at either end will cause elbow pain. Plus, standing too far from the stack will make your abs contract like crazy.

Once you have found a happy medium, contract the tricep slowly and throughout the whole movement. Try not to let the angle between your upper and lower arm bones get less than 90 degrees. That's about the limit of how far the tricep can be stretched before it gets relatively weaker. Some movement in the entire arm is actually fine, as long as you don't start looking like a church bell ringer.

Dumbbell lying tricep extension

Dumbbells are fairly easy to get into position for extensions, particularly if you use one arm at a time. They find their own groove nicely too. The only problem are the jumps in the dumbbells (weight wise), and lowering them too far.

Gym dumbbells tend to go up in big percentages on small movements. This is one area where home gym adjustable dumbbells have the edge. If you have cash to flash, and love the exercise, you could consider getting small magnetic weights that attach to most dumbbells. These are called "fractional plates" or "micro plates". They are expensive, but you could use them to make small but longer progress on other exercises too. If you find jumps too much, you could work in lower rep ranges for a while ('til your strength increases), or find another exercise. Some people can tolerate weight jumps more than others.

And the other problem as mentioned, is excess range of motion. Dumbbells become a victim of their own free-swinging success. If you lower them too far, i.e. bring your hand back so that the tricep tendon is heavily stretched, you could cause problems. A basic rule is if your tendons don't hurt, you're fine.

Sounds obvious, but you'd be surprised by how few pay attention to pain signals, and sometimes even just pop pills to get through it. By the way, if you ever find muscle soreness, enjoy it. Certainly don't take anti-inflammatory medication (e.g. *Advil* / *Nurofen*, both forms of ibuprofen) as they can block the natural muscle growth response.

Barbell lying tricep extension (EZ curl bar)

This exercise is a classic, and can produce great results. The only caution is about protecting your elbows. A straight bar *can* be used, but it takes experience, and a slightly strange "loose handshake" type grip. This takes lots of feel, which is especially difficult while maintaining tricep mind-muscle connection. For this reason, an EZ curl bar is preferred.

You can get into the start position yourself, but you may find it easier to get someone to hand the bar over. Even then, it's best if the person is experienced, and gives you time to nail the perfect grip before giving you the "your bar" signal.

If you have no one to spot you (or if you hate all the guys in the gym that day), bear in mind there will come a time when the weight is so heavy, getting it into place becomes an injury risk.

The main goal is to find an elbow position where they don't hurt at all. Because you are placing the whole tricep muscle in a stretched position, shifting a heavy weight might stress the main tendon. If this happens regardless of elbow placement, consider an exercise like pushdowns. We all vary in how much stretch our various tendons can take. Don't be upset if you find you have tight tendons. On the flip side, they mean you are more likely to generate high power due to strong *stretch-reflex* reactions.

Keep a looseness in the movement, in terms of not being obsessed with maintaining stillness of elbows. Many guys have a training partner hold their elbows in place. This is a bad idea. It's far better to let the elbows go from being slightly back (towards your head) at the start, and then gently gliding forwards as you contract to full extension. And again, ignore gym broscience about the need for constant tension. You can relax a bit at the top, especially if this helps you pre-set for the next rep.

ABDOMINALS

Hanging leg-raise

This is *not* an easy exercise, but it's the best if you can master it. The hanging variation is superior to one performed on a supported unit. Hanging encourages the spine to *decompress*, which is partly why it's so good. With a relaxed spine, the abs contract harder.

Hang from a bar which is high enough to have your feet avoid touching the ground. If you have no choice, at least find a bar where you can do it with bent knees.

A bent-knee raise is less effective, as your bent knees create a lighter "weight", but it's still decent.

The key is to raise your almost straight legs (a slight unlocking is natural) *as high as possible*. <u>At the minimum,</u> this means above parallel. Do not copy others who stop level, because at that point, your abs have mainly contracted isometrically (i.e. without changing length), and your hip flexors have worked concentrically (i.e. shortened). When you go *beyond* level, the abs begin to contract, and your pelvis (hip bone area) tilts backwards. Ideally, you get to the point where your feet reach your *head height*.

If you swing around between reps, you don't have enough ab strength yet. This is necessary to keep you still as the movement begins (so that the hip flexors can contract and lift your legs to the 90 degree level). Stick with it (even if it means using the Swiss ball to get strength in the meantime).

Swiss / stability ball crunch

Find a larger ball to start with (e.g. 65cm / 26"), as these are actually easiest for most people. Because the ball is big, the curve of your spine is less. That therefore means the stretch on your abs is not too much either. As you get better, work towards a smaller sized ball (e.g. around 50cm / 20"). A smaller ball means being "draped" over it more, and hence your abs will work harder.

The key to this exercise *is* to let your body drape, allowing it to stretch your abs. It's *not* a stability exercise, even if you find it that way in the beginning. It's about the abdominal wall getting a nice stretch so that it can get an equally nice contraction. Place your hands by your temples, and focus on breathing out as you come up. Most abdominal work is best performed by breathing out as you contract. The lack of air allows the abdominal muscle fibers to shorten maximally.

SPINE

Back extension

Without doubt, this is the most poorly performed exercise ever, with less than 1 in 300 having correct technique. **Back extensions are designed for your spinal muscles**, not hamstrings or glutes. If you're trying to hit glutes and hams, you need a different piece of kit (a *glute-ham developer*). Most trainee's back extensions look like stiff-legged deadlifts. Their hams and glutes stretch and contract, lifting and lowering their *whole* upper body. Meanwhile, their spinal muscles get a tiny pump from holding itself *almost straight*. Your spine is supposed to be the bit that lengthens and shortens! It's literally a crunch in reverse.

Correctly performed, the upper body moves *way* less. Set the bench so the supportive pad sits just below your hip bones. Touch your fingers to the sides of your head, or cover your face using your palms. Do not put your hands behind your head. Instead of a back movement, imagine you are upside down in space, and trying to do a crunch. This will lengthen your spinal muscles. Then, simply reverse. Start with the lower spine, then gradually contract the mid spine, the upper spine, and finish by looking up with your head. To start again, drop the head, then the upper spine, then the mid, and finally the lowest part. It's only one spine you have, but there's movement in 3 to 4 areas of it.

Your mobility depends on the quality of your mind-muscle connection. If you're having a problem visualizing this (and there aren't many decent training videos either), use the exercise below to get some feeling first.

Standing back roll (barbell / dumbbell)

This is similar to a back extension, with a less loaded range of movement. It can be done without equipment also. From a standing position, take a light barbell (i.e. a small fixed-weight barbell if possible) or two light dumbbells. Standing tall, gradually let the weight pull you forwards, as if you're bowing but without much movement at your hips. Feel the spine lengthen as you lean forward. At a *naturally* stretched limit, reverse the movement, gradually contracting the lower, mid and upper areas of the spine.

To help get a feel for this, do it without any external weight in the beginning. Start with a slight lean forwards, then drop the head, mid back, and lower back. Slowly reverse.

Imagine your spinal muscles lengthening and shortening like an accordion instrument. If you are still unsure of the technique, look up "actors spinal rolls" on the 'net.

DISCOURAGED EXERCISES

The previous chapters give enough variety to keep you happy for a while, but if you're fidgety, read this before heading elsewhere. What follows is a small list of potentially dangerous or useless exercises. You may disagree, especially if you've used them before without a problem. This *dirty dozen* <u>is</u> here for a reason. And, all of them have safer alternatives that you can push harder on, and for longer.

CHEST

Incline barbell / dumbbell press

Inclines *slightly* increase upper chest stimulation over using a flat bench. But they also substantially increase injury risk to the shoulders. We rarely push at this angle in nature. A low-incline (20 degrees or lower) is safer, but you may as well use a flat bench then.

The upper chest, also known as the *clavicular pectoral*, works heavily in flat bench work. It also works heavily in most overhead presses and raises. For example, the military press, an *almost* upright press, hits the upper pecs hard. Although it isn't an easy exercise, it's safer than the in-between angle we call *incline*.

Decline barbell / dumbbell press

Decline movements boost lower chest stimulation over the flat bench, but they're awkward to get in and out of.

While their range of motion and shoulder position is better than inclines, you can easily "fall off" the correct groove and put your shoulders at risk. And because of the high legs position, there's an off-putting head rush to deal with. On a heavy set with awkward breathing, it can feel like your head is going to explode. This distracts from optimal mind-muscle connection.

Dips (or dip machine) are a superior alternative. Next time you see someone do them in the gym, watch from the side. Then watch someone doing declines. They share a similar plane of motion, but dips allow better control, better mind-muscle connection, and less chance of a head rush.

Dumbbell flyes (any)

These create an excessive stretch at the end of the movement that eventually ruins shoulders. And there's always a strong temptation to stretch, because most of the dumbbell flye range of motion has weak resistance. This means you spend little time in the productive part, and too long in the stretch. Our shoulders aren't designed to be used that way.

We tend to naturally shorten the arm lever by bending it, making it almost like a press. Or we would use the flye motion but with less stretch, and use all our power around the contracted position (e.g. a hook punch).

A cable flye - *especially a standing one-armed version* - is safer and more productive.

LATS

Behind-the-neck pulldown or pull-up

These movements were popular in the 1970s, before we knew better, i.e. before years of doing them started to show up shoulder injuries. Unless you have *really* flexible shoulders, anything behind-the-neck is dangerous for their joints. Plus, there is not much benefit in terms of muscle alignment compared to pull-ups or pulldowns to the front.

Bent-over barbell row / free-standing T-bar row

These can be good, but the average guy will get equal benefit from a one-arm dumbbell row. Done poorly and to exhaustion, the bent-over barbell row puts your spine in a dangerous position. Most trainees have weak spinal muscles that cannot hold their upper body in place. The *supported* t-bar row is an excellent exercise, although some find the compression of their chest and breathing a problem.

SHOULDERS

Barbell upright row

The barbell fixes the path of the arms too rigidly, potentially damaging shoulders. Also, people tend to use too much weight, making it a forearm (*brachioradialis*) and arm flexor (*brachialis*) exercise. If they manage to work their shoulders, the path of the barbell limits the shoulder joint's free design.

Internally rotating the upper arm bones (turning them inward if viewed from above) can make them grind inside their space, gradually destroying them. Welcome to *Snap City!* Dumbbells are good if they're pulled along a natural line.

Behind-the-neck shoulder press

Again, a popular 1970s movement. Unfortunately, it forces shoulder joints into an unnatural position for 99% of trainees. Olympic lifters spend time developing extra flexibility in this area so they can perform other lifts. Most people are not Olympic lifters. Even when those guys take time off, they need to spend a while getting the range back. It's <u>not</u> natural for a human to be flexible in that area. Behind-the-neck presses also force the neck forward awkwardly. Finally, it's a nightmare movement to spot. Pressing to the front (i.e. military press) is a superior choice.

HAMSTRINGS

Stiff / Bent-leg / Romanian deadlift

These are highly difficult movements to perform safely. They require excellent spinal strength combined with intense mind-muscle connection. The Romanian Deadlift is not actually a dead-lift, as in it doesn't have a stop-start nature. Instead, it involves carefully controlled tension of hamstrings, spinal muscles and glutes.

It's impossible to recommend for most people, as the risk-to-reward ratio is in completely the wrong direction.

Good Mornings

This is effectively a stiff-legged deadlift while standing up. The pressure on the spine, both lower and upper (near the neck) is tremendous. This movement famously damaged the seemingly indestructible Bruce Lee, and took him out for 6 months. Work your hamstrings and low spine with safer movements for sure (leg curls and back extensions respectively). Or do them and get ready to say "Good morning doctor...".

TRICEPS

Tricep kickbacks (dumbbell, cable)

Kickbacks of any kind put the tricep in a completely unstretched and unnatural position. In this state, the triceps (or any unstretched muscle) cannot generate proper muscular tension. Some swear by the *feeling of being contracted*. In fact, it comes from the muscle being *so* slack that it's bunched up on itself. In addition, the way most people perform a kickback creates no resistance for most of the movement.

BICEPS

Reverse curl (barbell, dumbbell, cable, EZ curl bar)

Technically, reverse curls are not a bicep exercise. They proportionally hit the large forearm muscle, the *brachioradialis*, and the muscle under the bicep, the *brachialis*.

This curl variation puts the bicep tendon in an awkward position, and although it's not excessively risky, it focuses on muscles that nature never intended to use in complete isolation. This can cause tendon pain. It's also not necessary, as both brachialis and brachioradialis work hard during regular curls. If you're worried about not seeing the brachialis muscle on the side of your arm, this is partly genetic (in terms of how much to the *outside* your brachialis is positioned), and much to do with your overall body fat level. If you get to 12% body fat or less, you will see your brachialis. I bet it won't look neglected.

THIGHS

Deadlift

Of course I had to save the best for last, as in, the worst. You may think it's controversial, and copy what everyone says regarding "deads" being the best mass builder. To sweeten you up to my point of view, I admit that the deadlift hits a lot of meat. Your thighs, glutes, spine, traps and forearms all feel it. There is also an isometric contraction in the lats. But overall, it's thighs, butt and spine. Which you hit most depends on your structure: some get more thighs while others pull with the spine. Poor technique can vary what areas you hit too.

Regardless of your proportions, I advise against deadlifts. To call them a "basic exercise" is crazy, as there are so many parts to go wrong. This can even happen *during* a set that starts well. To perform them safely they need to be hit with low reps (e.g. 5). Sometimes doubles or triples work best (2 or 3 reps). This limits growth potential, unless you do a high number of sets. And in that case, you need sustained concentration to maintain form.

On traditional length sets (6 and above), tiredness kicks in and technique flies out of the window.

This turns the mass building poster boy into a recipe for disaster, potentially screwing up your training for months. Damage to the spine will limit your ability to push on *all* exercises, as there's no way to avoid using the body's central hinge.

Other injuries include overuse of the hip joints, and bicep tears when using a mixed grip (one hand over, one hand under). Even though the biceps are working isometrically - i.e. not changing length - they are vulnerable in an outstretched position. If you don't believe this, do a *YouTube* search and get ready to wince. The palm-up side usually snaps.

The squat is also not "basic", but it's much safer and more productive. The shrug / trap bar can be used to deadlift, although many call it a squat (some say *squat-lift*). It's a good movement. Because your hands are at your sides, you're not forced forward excessively. And when you're more upright, the spine is better protected.

******

So there you have it, the dirty dozen. Show them to your gym buddies if you like. You will meet people who swear by one or more of them. They might even have good gains from them. Regardless, they could have got equal or faster gains with other movements, and certainly done less wear and tear. Until you hear otherwise, ditch these dozen devils.

SECTION 2:
OUT OF THE GYM

EAT, EAT, AND EAT AGAIN

There's no way round this. To get *swole*, you need to eat more than most people. Actually with today's mega calorie world, in terms of pure *energy*, it might not be *more*. But you definitely need to pay more *attention* to your food. An Average Joe's main concern is filling their belly either when they feel hungry - or - when their partner, boss or schedule allows them to. You are not an Average Joe.

This chapter is a beast, but it's an interesting beast. And I go into detail so you can truly *understand* what you're doing. When you understand, you don't need to remember. This makes it easier to take positive daily actions, again and again. Some stuff might seem repetitive, but repetition makes an expert.

It's more important to get the message of this chapter right - *the structure of eating* **- than even <u>what</u> you eat.**

The human body can thrive all over our planet, in different climates and with different food supplies. It's an incredibly adaptive machine. But for getting swole - you must, must, *must* - get the <u>structure</u> correct. Amounts and type of food are relatively personal, and can vary lots *if* you get this other stuff down.

Don't be like 90% of trainees, who think they can cover diet with the occasional protein shake. That's BS. Your body is simply too smart to be cheated.

No human can defy the laws of biochemistry.

Your concerns about food need to be along these lines:

- the **timing** of meals
- the **frequency** of meals
- the **balance** of meals
- the **stickability** of meals

Let's deal with them in that order.

THE TIMING OF MEALS

There are times when food becomes *more* important, at least for guys who workout. They are:

- when you wake up
- before your workout
- after your workout
- before you sleep

IMPORTANT MEAL #1 - **WHEN YOU WAKE UP**

After you've slept, or should have slept, your body is slightly lower on nutrients. Throughout the night, your brain and other organs have been active. This is because during that time, most of the body enters *repair* mode. Skin cell production, for example, doubles during sleep. And of course, muscles continue to repair.

The brain is an energy intense organ, gobbling up 25% of your daily calories. As you sleep, it gets its preferred fuel - *glucose* - from the local glucose dealer: your liver. By the time morning comes, the liver is getting empty.

This can make you feel hungry first thing. If you ignore it, your body eventually shifts over to burning stored body fat. Sounds cool.

The problem is, somewhat depending on genes, it can also burn *muscle* in this state. Well, *burn* is the wrong term. It pulls protein out of your muscle and sends it to the liver - which tears it into "spare" parts like a vehicle breaker - creating glucose for your brain. Science calls this **gluconeogenesis**. I calls it annoying. Since your goal is to get swole, I wouldn't hang around to see if that's where your DNA takes you. Instead, I'd eat breakfast.

If swole is your goal, you can't skip breakfast.

If you've worked out close to bedtime the night before, you *really* need your morning munch. There are other times when skipping breakfast *is* useful, such as gunning for rapid fat loss or when using *intermittent fasting* to improve general health. But for getting futuristically swole, old fashioned *is* best. Meal one must happen when you wake up.

If by chance breakfast is the first meal before you workout, read the next bit, and tailor your choices around that. Final reminder:

Eat when you get up.

IMPORTANT MEAL #2 - **BEFORE YOU WORKOUT**

The meal before you hit the weights is often called your **pre-workout meal**. The phrase "pre-workout" now means supplements designed to boost your workout performance. Ironically, <u>no</u> pre-workout supp can give you the energy that eating correctly gives you.

In fact, most people need pre-workouts (supplements) *because* they eat so badly. As we'll see, there's nothing fancy about pre-workout supps.

They rely on micronutrients - combos of vitamins, minerals, herbs and stimulants - to give you a *brain* boost. In reality, the biggest energy comes from **macronutrients** - aka *macros* - carbs, proteins and fats. It may sound unsexy, but it's also true. And whatever your opinion, correct macros *are* the stuff that might actually *make* you sexy.

The last meal before working out is an incredibly personalized meal. What's that? The key thing about this serving of food is that it **must** make you **feel good**. What is feeling good? Again, that's personal.

Aim to eat whatever makes you feel in the best shape to *smash* your workout.

Science has tried to determine "perfect" pre-workout meals, and repeatedly come up with problems. Originally, the safe and somewhat samey suggestions were to have a low-fat, high carb, moderate protein meal around 2 hours before. While this worked for many, careful analysis of the research revealed too many variations. Some people liked it in the experiment but not outside of the lab. Others hated all textbook recommendations.

Because **food** is linked to our **emotions**, what you eat is very likely to affect exercise performance. So, whatever you eat in the meal before training - don't have anything that:

- makes you feel physically uncomfortable
- makes you feel depressed about not picking something nicer

Your pre-workout meal should make you *feel* good.

Once you've found what does that, you'll want to time it well. Don't panic if your timing goes out the window sometimes; stuff happens so just roll with it. Ideal timing is to **leave a 1 to 3 hour gap between finishing your food, and hitting the weights**. Less than 1 hour isn't dangerous, and it might not even make you feel stuffed. But 1 hour or more is ample time for most meals to get their nutrients into your bloodstream. While food in the system means you won't burn tons of body fat, it will mean your recovery gets a head start. Fast recovery is important when using frequent full-body workouts.

At the top end, **working out more than 3 hours after your last meal is a bad idea**. It's not dangerous, and there's probably some food left in your stomach. But by the time you train, the imbalance between taking and using could start bugging you. That is, you could get hungry. In itself, there's nothing wrong with hunger. But if you get distracted, and that's possible with full-body workouts, you *might* be tempted to slack off. You must give your workouts everything. Without *stimulating* growth, no food, supplement or even drug has reason to work.

SHUT UP AND GIVE ME 20

Although I've said this pre-workout meal should make you feel good, it is important to always include some protein in it. When I mentioned nutrients getting into the blood by the time you work out, the main ones you want are *amino acids*. These smaller parts of protein directly interact and respond to your muscle cells' nucleus, its brain. No matter what source your protein comes from, it always ends up in the bloodstream as tiny amino acids. There are many aminos used to build humans, 8 of which we call **essential amino acids**. Those 8 must be gotten from our plates or shakers. Unless you choose a *really* weird source of protein, you will have enough of a balance to do the job. But when it comes to the *amount*, listen up:

Try to get 20 grams of protein in the meal before you train. The source of your protein is not critical, but the amount is. 20 grams turns on muscle machinery and gives you the best chance of getting super swole *fast*.

Oh, and an important and unusual request:

Do not add *extra* vitamins, minerals or anti-oxidants to the meal taken before a workout.

Research shows these prevent the "good" damage needed to make your body adapt. Put simply, an excess of vitamins and minerals could block your muscles from growing. Do not take them in your post-workout meal either. Any other meal is fine (unless breakfast *is* your pre-workout meal, in which case take them later).

Eat 1 to 3 hours before training. Get 20 grams of protein in that meal.

IMPORTANT MEAL #3 - **AFTER YOUR WORKOUT**

Whatever the broscientists say, this *is* the most important meal. Training with weights creates an unusual demand on the body. A *not*-normal demand if you like. And not giving it nutrients at this time **definitely** slows progress. Definitely, definitely, definitely. You can skip the meal after your workout and burn more fat or improve other health factors - <u>but</u> - you will not get swole anywhere near as quick as if you EAT!

Cynical broscientists insist that the original advice to eat soon after workouts was driven by supplement companies wanting to make a profit. Of course they want to make a profit, they're companies! But that still doesn't mean eating after a workout is wrong. In fact your own body is keen to make a profit after training, and it certainly doesn't like creating a *loss*.

So, how soon should you eat after working out? As you put the squat bar back in the rack? While you're in shower? I need to be **very** specific:

One of your meals must be post-workout, and it should be taken between 15 and 30 minutes after your last rep.

Am I serious, *between* 15 and 30 minutes? Yes. Better say it again.

Eat between 15 and 30 minutes after working out. No sooner, no later.

Immediately after a workout isn't necessary, and in fact the body is *cooling down* even if you feel nothing. 15 minutes is enough time for blood flow to leave the last area you worked and re-distribute it around in a **normal** but *enhanced* pattern.

Beyond 30 minutes and your body starts to interpret the message you're sending it. Your message will say: I know I just worked you hard, but you're getting nothing. Go to bed, RIGHT NOW! This angry parent routine doesn't cut it with the body. It can start to break down muscle, sending it to the liver again, for disassembly and conversion to the body's master: the brain. It will also try to burn stored body fat as fuel, not a bad thing itself, but slow. Fat is like a solid log in the fire, and it needs lots of oxygen to burn (i.e. a whole day's worth).

In the meantime, damage starts to accumulate in the muscle tissue. While some damage *is* great, you want to limit that to damage stimulated **during** your workout.

Continuing damage due to underfeeding is bad news. Your next workout will suffer, meaning you spend less time growing. If you have a tough workout, and don't eat for ages, you'll see what I mean. You'll be sore the next day, a sign of deep, unhealed muscular damage. Because *Super Swole* involves frequent workouts, this kind of damage should be avoided.

Your goal is to stimulate - *recover fully* - and repeat. Multiple, *small* doses of muscular stimulation. To do this, you <u>must</u> recover quickly after *each* workout.

Waiting more than 30 minutes could edge you into the danger zone. If you leave it too long, your body assumes no food is coming and decides to help itself. The net result is that your hunger might turn off for a bit (while it eats body fat and muscle) putting you at more risk. It might eventually make you sleepy.

By the way, you want your post-workout meal to be liquid. Yes, there is *some* research showing not much difference between a solid meal and a liquid one. In - a - lab! The real world is different. I've already said you need to eat between 15 and 30 minutes after your workout. A solid meal at this time makes it harder. You either have to bring it with you to the gym or wait on someone to serve it.

The natural desire after a workout is to drink, not physically chew. Considering a liquid meal contains more - ahem, liquid - than a solid meal, you get the benefit of rehydration. And a fully hydrated muscle cell is more *anabolic* than a dehydrated one. So, go for liquid. Of course this limits your options, which is why there's a chapter on the post-workout meal coming up.

For now, here's your summary:

Consume a liquid meal, between 15 and 30 minutes after working out. Consult the section on post-workout meal for what to put in it, and how much.

IMPORTANT MEAL #4 - **BEFORE YOU SLEEP**

As discussed earlier, sleep is *active*. Stuff gets repaired. Eating immediately before bed isn't a great idea, mainly because the physical discomfort in your belly makes drifting off hard (at least in healthy guys). Also, blood sugar spikes after eating *might* reduce the burst of growth hormone that hits 90 minutes after nodding off. Beyond a certain blood sugar level, growth hormone struggles to rise. Repeatedly blocking nature's rhythm is destructive to your skin, tendons, recovery and overall health.

Having said all this, **you shouldn't go to sleep on empty**, at least not if you're aiming for swoledom. An entirely empty belly makes it hard to sleep because you're likely to be aware of feeling hungry. And getting anxious means not getting any kip.

Most importantly, you want a *trickle* of late night nutrients to be available. This combination of nature's planned downtime, adequate repair materials, and you not making any physical demands, creates the perfect environment for muscular growth.

Aim to eat this final meal so that you finish with at least **one hour before you lay down**. This gives your body some space to get rid of excess liquid, making a comfortable, uninterrupted sleep more likely.

It's also the minimum period with which your stomach can make progress in liquidizing whatever you've chucked down the pipe. Again, this makes the physical comfort of sleep more achievable. At the same time:

Don't leave more than a 3-hour gap between putting your fork down and putting your head down.

Although your stomach is not technically "empty" after 3 hours, stretch receptors around it might make you *feel* that way. This could make you edgy. Remember, you are not an Average Joe, and your training increases your body's attention towards how you feed it after being attacked (the workout). More than 3 hours means that some portion of your sleep-recovery will suffer from a lack of nutrient flow. In a normal person, this is not a problem. In fact, it's probably healthy. But you're not a normal person, and you don't aspire to have a normal person's *body*. Your training places above average demands on it, and your dietary habits must change accordingly. **Your dietary habits must be above average.**

THE FREQUENCY OF MEALS

Bodybuilders have been banging on about the need to eat frequent meals for years. Their attitudes towards meal frequency first spread to athletes, and then finally infected the general public. That's right, *infected*. The idea with small, frequent meals - in a health sense - is that your blood sugar remains stable, compared to eating fewer but bigger meals. Also, the theory is that small meals ramp up your metabolism, and keep you slim. It's true, *in theory*. If you divided your normal meals into smaller portions, spreading them out, you might add less fat to your hips. The reason? A tiny bit of each meal's digestion is actually *spent* on the digestion process itself.

But here's reality: when you ask people to eat smaller, more frequent meals, they just eat **more meals**! More calories, more sugar, more fat, and who knows what else.

As for average blood sugar levels, they remain higher too. Epic fail. But what about gaining muscle? Hitting the weights definitely increases the demands on the body. In a way, it puts you back to being a baby again, as you're suddenly growing once more. Remember, unless you train, your body has a strong tendency to stay *exactly* the same. But stimulate growth, and it can't just build a new body from thin air. We literally are what we eat. Competitive bodybuilders still take on 5 to 12 meals per day. But is it overkill? Absolutely. And for many reasons.

PROBLEMS WITH 5 MEALS AND ABOVE

You feel like you're always eating! Seriously, that's no joke. We all have 24 hours in a day, and spend two-thirds of that awake. After you take out time for getting dressed, showering and travelling, the consumption of 5 meals and beyond becomes **stressful**. If you study or have a job, eating that frequently might be impossible without you getting sneaky. That's more pressure, and more chance of attracting general criticism from those around you. While I don't suggest you simply fold when people push your buttons, I also say: don't *look* for trouble.

Eating 5 meals and above also means more cost, more time spent preparing, and the real killer, more **boredom**. This last point is important, especially if you want to keep up the consistency required for serious muscle gain. Avoid boredom in any long-term plan.

PROBLEMS WITH 3 MEALS AND BELOW

There's too much pressure on each meal. Pressure on a meal? With just three bites at the cherry, each meal has to cram in enough protein, energy, fat, carbs, fiber, and enjoyability.

That alone might make those meals uncomfortable, either physically for your digestion, or mentally in terms of you needing to tick nutrient boxes.

Three meals or less, the classic *breakfast, lunch and dinner* also means there will be **lengthy gaps** between fuel stops. In an Average Joe, this isn't a problem. Just grab a snack to keep you going, be it an "energy" drink, cookies, or pizza. This *is* a problem for someone wanting to get in amazing shape. Eating excess food adds body fat, covering all your hard earned muscular gains, making you actually appear *smaller* (when the shirt's off).

Excess body fat lowers *average* testosterone. Body fat also contains an enzyme called *aromatase*. This converts whatever testosterone you have left into the hormone **estrogen**. And estrogen only makes one part of you swole (your nips!). There are aromatase-blocking supplements and drugs, but none compare to being in-shape. **Keep lean, keep testosterone**.

The long gaps between 3 meals or less also tempt you off the consistent healthy-eating path. Such bad habits tend to partner up with more bad habits (more about this in *the stickability of meals*). In a nutshell, if you eat too infrequently - and then reach for junk - you might start making your *whole lifestyle* junk also. So, what's left? You do the math!

EAT 4 TIMES PER DAY

After years of witnessing *every* combination of meal timing and frequency, this is what you need to know:

Four meals per day is optimal for gaining muscle.

It is the *Goldilocks* amount. Not too much, not too little. Four meals allows you to evenly spread your calories, protein, carbs and fat. It prevents hunger from rising (i.e. prevents you reaching for Average Joe food), and it's not so frequent to make you feel anti-social or trapped on a merry-go-round. Plus, you can make one of these feedings your **post workout meal**.

Ideally, spread the 4 meals roughly apart. I said *roughly* because *life* is rough. You'll have days where your schedule changes slightly, or where your appetite doesn't like obeying the clock. This is normal, and you should roll with it. That's another reason why 4 is optimal; there's leeway to shift meals around and still not end up too close together, or drift too far apart. **Eat four times per day**. 'Nuff said.

THE BALANCE OF MEALS

By balance, I mean **no meal - with perhaps *one* exception - should be made up of just a single macro** (macronutrient). Put simply, every meal should contain *some* protein, *some* carbs and *some* fat. Remember, this advice is specifically geared to getting swole. It's not middle-of-the-road general advice. What's so special about a balance of macros? Consistency. There it is again. To ensure a *steady flow of nutrients*, and importantly a *steady flowing mind*, balanced macros always beat out other combos long-term.

BAD COMPANY

There are times when low-carb meals work, or no-carb meals, like protein with fat. And, there are times when high protein and high carb meals with *no* fat work (more about this in a sec). But generally, these are for specialized results, such as losing fat fast.

There is <u>no</u> reason to combine *high fat* and *high carb*.

Well, unless your dream is to quickly become a sumo wrestler. This particular combo guarantees body fat gain. High carbs raise insulin, the hormone that stores everything away, and high fat (especially high saturated fat - take note paleo hacks) is easily converted *into* body fat itself. With high insulin opening up your body fat cell doors, and high dietary fat willing to step inside, you create a perfect storm for weight gain. The worst possible food for this? French fries. Research actually backs this up, with fries topping *all* foods in terms of actual body fat gained per portion of food eaten. I mean, they literally studied fat being deposited *while it happened*. Pizza was second.

Back to the main point, your meals must strive for balance. Treat the macros of protein, fat and carbs equally. When it comes to protein, research has tested different types of regimes. It's tried to give people a huge amount of protein in one meal, called *pulse* feeding. And, it's tried giving it over many meals (16!). This is called *spread* feeding. The results have gone in both directions, depending on who the subjects were. For example, in older women, the benefits of enhanced protein synthesis were strongest if they had *one* serving of protein at midday.

If they took the same amount and spread it out, there wasn't much of an anabolic effect. In young guys, this pattern didn't work.

We now understand that when it worked, it didn't happen because the body prefers protein at one meal only, but because tiny protein meals didn't have *enough* in each one to trigger the body's muscle building "machinery". As some people get older, they need a bigger shot of protein to create the anabolic effect.

Recent research actually used people who work out regularly. Without doubt, results show **evenly spread out meals work best**.

Later on, when you find out how much protein you need in total, try dividing it into *roughly* equal doses (like a medicine). The amount of carbs should be linked to your need for energy. Fats usually take care of themselves, but as you'll see, there are some you might want to *add* a bit of.

THE EXCEPTION

Post-workout, it's fine to have a technically unbalanced meal. You'll try to exclude fat of any kind (mono, unsaturated, saturated *and* essential fat). Fat slows down the transport of food through the digestive system, and it's the one time you want super efficient digestion. Also, fat of any kind, temporarily reduces arterial blood flow. Again, post-workout is a period you cannot afford that. Your arteries are highways for nutrient delivery, and you want them as *fast flowing* as possible. The better you recover from your workout, the better your next one will be.

THE STICKABILITY OF MEALS

You don't think that's a word do you? But you get what it means. Meals have to be enjoyable, and they have to be repeatable. Very few meals, and very few people, can combine these two factors. Anyone can eat an enjoyable meal, but ask them to eat it multiple times per week, and it starts to test their sanity. In short, it stops being enjoyable, and obviously that's not easy to *stick* with. **Find stickability**.

I'll say it again. You need to find meals - that's combinations of foods - that you enjoy *and* don't mind repeating. There will be some compromise of course.

As in, these meals might not be 10 out of 10 in enjoyability, but they should have *enough* in them to keep you coming back for more, even if you have to see the usual suspects *again* tomorrow. Why is this important? **Routine works**. Consistent eating yields consistent results. It's equally important as training and other factors.

The relationship between what you eat, how you train, and how motivated you feel, is completely linked.

And it's linked in every direction. If you train well, you will be tempted to eat better. If you eat better, you will be tempted to train smartly. Of course the flip side exists also. If you skip some training, you'll probably reach for junk. And if you eat junk, you'll just go through the motions in the gym next time. It's this relationship that makes eating consistently decent food, *so* important. Now you can see why meals with high stickability increase your general rate of success.

When you eat like this, be prepared for some resistance, especially in the criticism and confusion from your non-training friends or family. They will tell you your diet is boring, stupid, and not social. They might even tell you to stop.

Do not give up your dreams just to fit someone else's idea of "food". Many people, family, friends and even loved ones see your determination, and fear being left behind.

Be polite with any criticism, say "maybe", and then do what you were doing anyway. As Muhammad Ali once said, *nothing tastes as good as lean and mean feels*. Find stickability in most of your meals, and you will be mastering your diet.

Well done on getting through this. If you understand what you've just read, you will be more advanced than 99% of gym trainees (and their trainers). *What* you eat is discussed often, but *how* you eat is most important.

The structure and timing of your food is crucial. More crucial than what's actually in the meals.

Now you know that, let's get some more specifics done.

BRO VS PRO

bro

- ✗ you need to eat 6 meals a day
- ✗ just eat normally and you'll be fine
- ✗ forget food before training, just take pre-workouts

pro

- ✓ eat 4 meals per day, roughly spaced apart
- ✓ meal timing and meal stickability are very important
- ✓ you cannot eat like an Average Joe if you want to get swole

PROTEIN - THE SIMPLE TRUTH

Now you have your meal structure sorted, you'll want to know what to put in them. Let's start with protein. After all, the word itself means "of first importance" in ancient Greek. Protein is the most endlessly debated macronutrient in forums, videos and gyms. By the way, a macronutrient - or *macro* - is just a name given to the 5 big nutrients that make up the human diet. The other four are fat, carbs, water and fiber. When it comes to protein, **the truth is simple**. You need to:

- **have more** than Average Joe
- **time it** better than Average Joe

That's the basics. Let's break it down a bit further.

HAVE MORE THAN AVERAGE JOE

Why? Because you're not average, especially if you're adding lots of muscle in a short period of time. Left alone, your body wants to stay the same. That's the safest, most economical thing for it to do. By hitting the gym, especially with full-body workouts, you are rapidly increasing the rate of protein turnover, i.e. the balance between what's coming in through **dietary protein**, and what's being broken down in **body protein**. You want to be in a *slight* positive balance. Excess protein will be processed by the kidneys, added as body fat (unlikely), or lost through extra heat production.

Muscles, apart from being water, are mainly protein. In fact, if you took all the water out of the human body, **half of what's left would be protein**. The rest would be minerals (bones), fat (including your brain), and a small amount of carbs (stored in the liver and muscles). Protein is being added or subtracted from the body constantly, and it's your job to *tip* the balance in favor of being added. By training correctly, with intense mind-muscle connection, you will stimulate the demand to add protein. You then must keep the other side of the deal, by feeding your body the raw materials. Your body can make fats, and it can even make carbs, but it cannot make proteins. At best, it can recycle proteins from one area to another - from muscle to organs, organs to muscle, and muscles to muscles - but this is not actual *growth*. It's desperation. And a desperate body *looks* desperate.

ENOUGH IS ENOUGH

So, how much is enough? Average Joe gets by on 0.36 grams of protein per pound of bodyweight (or 0.8 grams of protein per kilo). If Average Joe was fighting Floyd Mayweather for the welterweight boxing title, he'd need just 53 grams of protein. Of course, if I was Average Joe, I wouldn't step into the ring with that kind of nutrition. These government figures were calculated to be effective for 99% of the population. In theory, it contains an in-built safety margin to cover active people. Except it doesn't really. The figures are old, and even newer versions don't do healthy guys justice. Especially those with *swole* aspirations.

Recent studies - using people who train - show that up to 0.8g of protein per pound of bodyweight is useful (1.8g per kg).

Beyond this amount, there is no clear benefit.

For example, if you were taking on Floyd for the same welterweight title, you'd be smarter taking in 120 grams instead of Average Joe's 53. And while we talk boxing, don't think today's champs survive by occasionally glugging down Rocky Balboa's five morning eggs in a glass (although that is a decent amount of a decent protein). Their protein intake is *precise*.

The old standard of 1 gram protein per pound of bodyweight (2.2g per kilo) sounds neat, but it's too much. You might say, "it's only a bit more". Well, only a bit more *is* a bit more than you need. It's more expensive for you, for the planet, and it may reduce gains by *displacing* other food in the diet. You see, protein is extremely effective at reducing appetite. If you eat too much, some will be turned into glucose, and you may never find the urge to eat other swole promoting foods. Foods that contain phytochemicals (plant chemicals, good ones), fiber, carbs and essential fats. If you've ever dieted and cut out a particular food, you may notice that later in the day, your body makes up for it by sneakily making you overeat something else. The only way to fight these "set-points" is to gradually lower them. Trust me, your body is the greatest guard dog ever seen, and if you try to get past it without obeying the rules, it will bark, and eventually bite. So, stick to a max of 0.8 grams of protein per pound of bodyweight (1.8 grams per kilo).

TIME IT BETTER THAN AVERAGE JOE

In addition to getting more, you need to time it better. By now, you should understand the need to spread it out. Remember, we found 4 key times to eat. Upon waking, before our workout, after our workout, and before bed. Each of these meals should contain some protein. By doing that, you achieve a couple of things:

- you turn on muscle building mechanisms
- you shut down muscle breakdown mechanisms

Because the body can't *store* protein, dividing it up makes sense anyway. Actually it can store protein in a sense, by building muscle. Studies show that spreading protein equally is best. Because we aim to eat 4 times a day, there'll be a nice balance between having *enough*, and having it *often enough*. If the figures confuse you, here's an easy rough reminder:

Get 8 grams of protein for every 10 pounds you weigh.

or if you use the metric weight system...

Get 9 grams of protein for every 5 kilos you weigh.

These guidelines are for *every* day. You'll be using full-body routines that hit every muscle. Studies show there's an enhanced level of protein synthesis - that's building up muscle protein - for up to 48 hours after a workout. If you train every other day, you'll *constantly* be stimulating growth. Even if you train once every third day, you'll be growing for at least 2 days our of three. Therefore, there isn't an "off day" for your body's muscle building machinery, and hence you need to keep it stocked up.

On non-training days, you must still hit protein goals.

On those non-training days, you can divide your daily protein intake into *roughly* equal servings. It doesn't have to be exact. Just make sure by midnight, you've hit the total target. On training days, you should ideally put a good-sized chunk of protein into the post-workout meal.

This will mean there's a little less in all your other meals. We'll talk about that later. For now, I just want you to know that the daily total is the key number.

TOTALLY MISSED THE POINT?

By now, the keen ones amongst you might be asking, "okay, I know I have to hit my protein totals, but what about protein quality?". Actually, new studies tend to show that if you get *enough* protein, your body can grow adequately. It's the total amount which most people find difficult. Even on vegan diets - traditionally regarded as having the lowest quality proteins - there comes a point where it's the *total* being hit which determines whether muscle growth occurs (or not).

Protein quality, that's grams of protein retained by the body compared to the grams you take in, is slightly higher in animal based foods. In protein balance studies, they use mixed diets. In theory this means that by exclusively living on high quality proteins (e.g. whey), you may be able to grow on less protein *in total*. There's no proof of this concept in research (yet), so we have to assume, yet again, it's about hitting the daily total.

POST-WORKOUT PROTEIN QUALITY

The protein quality taken in just after training does seem to matter. It's almost certainly due to the urgency of the demands at that time.

Again, in theory, if you had enough of even a low-quality protein, you'd still grow. The problem with low-quality proteins, is that they're usually bulky, and bulky things don't go down well after a workout. As I said, there's more on post-workout protein selection soon.

For now, be aware of protein quality, but focus on hitting your daily totals. If you do that day after day, you'll notice that muscle growth shoots through the roof. Most trainees know they need protein, but very, *very* few actually do something about it.

It's interesting to note that when taking anabolic steroids, protein synthesis increases. That's an increase in muscle protein laid down. It does this through many mechanisms, one of which includes the body getting *more* from the protein you give it. Basically, the body becomes very efficient at absorption. But there's still a limit, and even a steroid user cannot create muscle from thin air. Many first time users notice some gains on steroids, but not in the amounts they imagined. And the reason is simple: they can't keep up with the increased demand for dietary protein. No drug on the planet can get you off your behind and make you take your protein.

You must make the effort - repeatedly - to hit your daily protein goals. If you do this, gains become easy.

Time for a little bro vs pro.

BRO VS PRO

bro

× just eat tons of meat every day
× get 1 gram of protein per pound
× protein quality is all that really matters

pro

✓ get 8 grams of protein per 10lbs of weight (9g per 5kg)
✓ spread your protein out evenly whenever possible
✓ make hitting your daily protein totals your priority

FATS AND FICTION

You might think it's strange, but there's good reason to talk about dietary fat when it comes to getting swole fast. Like many things in nature, it's important to strike the right balance. Specifically, you need to focus on *getting* two things:

- monounsaturated fat
- essential fats

Let's deal with monounsaturates first.

YOU SEXY MUFAs

Monounsaturated fats - abbreviated to MUFAs - are fats that are liquid at room temperature due to their chemical structure. Common sources include olive oil, sunflower oil, plus some meat and dairy products. Studies of athletes have shown that when monounsaturated (or saturated) fats are consumed, there's a positive association with testosterone. Simply said, when you eat or drink enough monounsaturated fat, testosterone seems to be higher *than when you don't*. On ultra-low fat diets, testosterone seems to be lower. Now, as all good scientists say - correlation doesn't prove causation - a fancy way of stating *just because you catch someone red-handed, doesn't mean they did it*. In the case of monounsaturates, it does seem there is proof though. Compounds found in olive oil, our best source of MUFAs, stimulate the testes to produce more testosterone. And remember, *your average level of testosterone is linked to your gains*. The higher it is, the easier it is to get swole.

Diets with low monounsaturates or saturates tend to churn out lower testosterone. While we keep mentioning saturated fats, you must be correctly informed about their downsides, which we'll discuss in a bit. For now, just make sure you get some monounsaturates in your diet. The easiest way?

OIL CHANGE

Olive oil is a widely available oil. As the olive is actually a fruit, it makes olive oil rare amongst oils, which generally come from seeds. The type of oil you want is **extra virgin olive oil**. This is the only oil that legally must be taken from good olives, during the early olive harvest, and extracted by old-fashioned *mechanical* means. This means grinding them between stones and squeezing all the oil out. Going old school means you keep the temperature down, and guarantee the oil's quality from field to plate.

Regular "olive oil" can be made from the worst olives, the bruised ones. Bruising means they've lost much of their nutrition. Try and buy oils from a well-known company. Producers have been caught out by government agencies that realized some were sneaking cheap oil into expensive bottles.

If you have any oils like sunflower, safflower, rapeseed or canola in your diet, start doing an oil change, i.e. swap them out in favor of extra virgin olive oil. You can only cook with olive oil on a low to medium heat, because after that it starts to smoke. Ideally, you shouldn't cook with *any* oil, as heat damages their structure. You can of course cook using different methods, like steaming or baking, and then add olive oil later. This is especially perfect for salads. Just add vinegar and some lemon juice, and you've got a classic, healthy, testosterone boosting dressing. And if you're not into adding oils in that way, here's the alternative.

During *Super Swole*, I suggest you take one to two tablespoons every day (15 to 30 mls). Use a little plastic measuring cup, and down it quickly with some liquid (e.g. a protein shake).

Extra virgin olive oil seems to protect the heart from damage. Remember, olives *are* fruit, and like most fruit, olives contain *anti-oxidants*. They're like dry paper towels, mopping up the water which causes rust damage on metal. Downing a small amount of neat extra virgin olive oil at least once a day is good for gains.

You can add extra virgin olive oil to any meal (apart from the post-workout meal). It adds calories and *satiety*. This simply means how *satisfied* you feel. Science has found that fat in food tends to make us feel more full and generally happier. In that state, you're less likely to snack. Don't overdo it though; **a tablespoon of extra virgin olive oil twice a day should be your limit**. The other half of high testosterone is keeping what you already have, and *that* is achieved by being lean (body fat contains enzymes which convert testosterone into the female hormone *estrogen*). What about those saturates?

THE SATS THAT FAIL YOU

Saturated fats have had quite a nutritional ride. First they were devils, being linked to heart disease, and then they were heroes, especially in the eyes of those who choose a caveman style of eating (so-called "paleo"). As mentioned just before, science has found that sat fats are positively linked with testosterone, i.e. if you eat more of them, you tend to have higher testosterone. You may also recall, I suggested you *don't* seek them out. Here's why (cavemen, shut your hairy ears):

Decreased blood flow - saturated fats reduce the way your artery walls perform. Instead of being all bouncy and flexible, they tend to be <u>stunned</u> after meals containing sat fats.

This isn't ideal for anyone, but if you're into training, it's especially annoying to not get a good pump. It's also annoying to get a heart attack when posing.

Decreased insulin sensitivity - Insulin is the body's storage hormone, needed to shuttle stuff into cells. For you, that includes amino acids, carbs, and even creatine. Sat fats reduce insulin's effectiveness, therefore reducing nutrient delivery to your biceps and pecs. Not ideal.

They make you fat! - In recent years, sat fats have been embraced by followers of the *Atkins Diet* and by paleo eaters. To make sat fats work well, you **must** follow an almost zero-carb diet. That's live off fats and protein, and nothing else. The *minute* you add carbs, sat fats cause chaos. You may have noticed that saturated fats are solid at room temperature. They are the white bits on meat, the grease in your eggs, and the hidden taste secret in your "healthy" salad dressing. The problem is, not all fat is equal in terms of being able to be burned as a fuel. In fact, **sat fats are the worst for burning**, i.e. they are the dietary fats stored most easily *as* body fat. And, they are the hardest to shift once inside you.

While many "weight-gain" programs don't care about weight-gain quality, I do. **We are not here to gain body fat**. It will make you look less muscular overall, and physiologically, excess body fat destroys your testosterone. As mentioned repeatedly, stored body fat contains *aromatase*, an enzyme that converts your man juice into estrogen. And too much estrogen will stop you getting swole. The old system of bulking and cutting came from a time before we could even *measure* hormones. Being fat is depressing, dangerous to health, creates stretch marks, and makes you look anything but an athlete.

So there are three strong reasons for you to avoid foods that are high in saturated fat. Next time you visit the store, walk past the extra virgin coconut oil (sat fat *extreme*), and pick up some good extra virgin olive oil instead. Is there any more on the topic? Yes, another few fats can *help*.

ESSENTIAL HELPERS

There are many different kinds of fat in nature, but technically, we need just two. When I say need, I mean if you don't ever get them, you'll eventually die, or at least *fail to thrive*. These are the appropriately named **essential fats**, *omega 6* and *omega 3*. They form the walls of most cells in your body, become part of your nervous system, improve circulation, and they can dramatically influence your immune reactions. In fact, the list of things they do is huge, and definitely beyond a book on getting swole. If you don't get enough of the essential fats, you may experience health problems. In *Super Swole*, those problems would be sore muscles and joints, and perhaps less of a pump during workouts (essential fats make arteries flow freely).

Essential fats are technically *polyunsaturates*, the third class of fats. They are very runny at room temperature, and react so much with air, that you need to keep them cool to prevent them going "off". This is why fish, rich in polyunsaturated fat, quickly becomes "rancid". That smell is the fats after they've reacted (think *rusted*) with oxygen. It's disgusting to our senses in order that we don't eat damaged fat. Clever really. Research has shown that while sat fats and monounsaturated fats help testosterone, *too much* polyunsaturated fat *lowers* it. It's unlikely you'd ever eat too much poly fat, unless you lived on fish (e.g. the Japanese) and swigged lots of vegetable oil (also a source of polyunsaturates).

How much omega 3 you need depends on your government. The *American Heart Association* thinks you should get 3 portions of oily fish per week (salmon, mackerel, trout), "natural" sources of omega 3. European authorities say you need a daily quarter gram of EPA and DHA, the two final chemicals that essential fats turn into. The Japanese scientists go for a percentage, stating roughly 3 to 4% of your calories should come from omega 3 and 6 fats.

By the way, omega 6 fats tend to get around. You'll find them in most oils, nuts and dairy. You don't need to *actively* seek them. But omega 3s, you might. If you regularly eat fatty fish, you should be fine. If you don't, it's best to get an omega 3 supplement. At most, you need something with **half a gram (500mg) of DHA or EPA** in it. EPA and DHA are the final types of omega 3 that the body needs.

Take omega 3 supplements at night (and definitely not in the post-workout meal). As they reduce inflammation, they can ease aches and pains, and help you wake up less sore.

Vegetarians and vegans can take supplements and don't need to be limited by fish oil capsules. In fact, fish don't produce *any* omega 3. They only have it because *they* eat plankton (plants which grow in the sea), and plankton make omega 3s in the first place. The fish eat the plankton, and people eat the fish. Ancient cavemen took it a step further when they ate the brains of humans (i.e. successful fishermen!). We can now produce pure DHA and EPA without going near a fish or a fisherman. It's actually the purest type of omega 3 available.

NEVER take more than 1 gram *total* of EPA / DHA per day. Studies show that it can suppress the immune system. And, an excess of polyunsaturates is linked to *lower* testosterone.

So there you have it, a basic rundown on dietary fat. Yes, you need some, but apart from a tablespoon or two of extra virgin olive oil, and maybe some omega 3, don't go seeking fat out. **High fat diets, in the presence of carbs, *make* you fat, and ultra low-fat diets *lower* your testosterone.** Just pick natural, moderate fat foods that you enjoy eating.

BRO VS PRO

bro

- ✕ just eat everything you can bro, including fat
- ✕ bulk up fast and cut down for summer
- ✕ high fat diets help everyone get shredded

pro

- ✓ add a bit of extra virgin olive oil and omega 3 to your diet
- ✓ avoid seeking out saturated fats if you want to be athletic
- ✓ eat natural foods in moderation and fat takes care of itself

CARBS - FRIEND OR FOE

Out of the 3 macros, carbohydrates are often the most debated, and definitely the most complicated. Protein and fat can be complex, but they generally fit into neat little boxes. There's the high protein / low protein camps, and high fat / low fat approaches. Simples. Carbs on the other hand, have people going to war over them. We have classic high carb / low carb debates, the glycemic index, discussion of what's paleo-friendly, talk of deadly fructose, the IIFYM (*if it fits your macros*) crowd, the percentages people, and those who love counting everything. So, where do we stand on carbs, especially in the context of *Super Swole*? Well before the specific advice, let's consider the things you can actually ignore.

COUNTING

Quite often in advice about gaining muscle, there's an emphasis on gaining *weight*. As you know, this isn't my thing. Gaining weight happens when you take in more than you take out, and there are endless ways to do that. The majority of today's adult population are masters of gaining weight, and they certainly don't need advice on doing it better. Considering most guys who want to gain muscle are secretly saying "I want to look good naked", it's shocking to see how much advice emphasizes *calories*. Trust me, if you want to look good in your birthday suit, it's not just about shoving more in.

There are also all kinds of carb-heavy formulas, like the advice to eat 16 calories per pound of bodyweight, or the more shocking, "eat 10,000 calories a day". Although eating excess calories is easy to start with, eating 10,000 a day becomes very difficult (not to mention, very expensive). And of course, it's ridiculous.

Counting calories, in a positive *eat at least this much to gain that* sense, is as pointless as going negative to lose weight. It never works out that simple. Adding calories generally means adding carbs, and usually adding fat. Excess in either is bad, but combined they're deadly. Eating a huge excess of carbs to big up your calories - no matter how healthy their origins - is destructive to health. The body fat gained lowers your useful testosterone, makes you sluggish, raises your disease risk, and makes you look like crap. So straight up, you can permanently forget about counting cals. And if you still have your calculator out...

(DON'T) DO THE MATH

The next common carb advice is to use percentages or count grams. I have recommended *grams of protein*, but that's appropriate. Without a minimum level of building materials (amino acids), growth is slow, if at all. With regards our dietary fat chat, I suggested just picking healthy foods, knowing that some fat would always hitch a ride. I mentioned a tablespoon or two of extra virgin olive oil, and perhaps adding some omega 3s. These are all do-able, becoming second nature habits within days.

However, when it comes to carbohydrates, I don't recommend counting grams. You already take care of protein, and doing it with carbs is a headache. Meals would become math, and that's no recipe for stickability. The same goes for percentages. I'm experienced in calculating facts about food, yet I'd struggle sticking to *percent of daily intake* guidelines. Those ratios are awkward for protein and fat too. If for example, I recommended you eat a 40/40/20 mix (carbs/fat/protein), you might manage it for a day. By day two, you'd be confused, fed up, and looking around for an alternative plan. Imagine a friend asking to get food with you. Could you honestly calculate individual proportions *on-the-fly*, and constantly re-evaluate your entire day, *just* to keep those "magic" percentages?

It's an impractical idea, first popularized by dietitians, and then by the governments they advised. The public has ignored percentages and specific *by the gram* recommendations for macros, because they're just too fiddly. Right, forget complex mathematical approaches to carbs. They don't fit life.

******

Before we go on, I need to address the wise guys who ask, "do we even need carbs?". The honest and *technical* answer is: no. Your body must have *essential* amino acids (protein), and it must have *essential* fats (omega 3 and 6). Other than that, we just need water, oxygen, sunlight and a long vitamin / mineral mix. There are no *essential* carbohydrates. We can make carbs from protein (including our own muscles), and even fuel our brain, heart and biceps from body fat (via a process called *ketosis*). In fact around the world, people thrive on many diets, all with varying amounts of carbs, or no real carbs at all (e.g. traditional *Eskimos*).

But this book is not just about surviving. It's called *Super Swole* for obvious reason. Getting swole, at least to the extent you want, isn't natural. It's natural to be lightly-built, athletic, and healthy, but swole is a modern invention. Cavemen did *not* have 16" arms! If you understand that, you'll hopefully accept that we need more than just a survival diet.

We need carbs to get swole.

FILL HER UP

Carbs easily replace glycogen, carbohydrate stores *inside* your muscle. This is crucial fuel for high-volume, high frequency full-body workouts.

These workouts are required for getting bigger. A zero carb or low-carb diet can work for many things, but they cannot power *this* muscle-building schedule.

PUMPING WATER

With the glycogen, carbs attract and store *intra-muscular* water. This hydration of muscle cells is good for growth itself, and it also ensures a good pump. A good pump ensures strong mind-muscle connection. And a strong mind-muscle connection promotes gains in size, instead of all-out strength.

FOOD FOR THOUGHT

Carbs also *reliably* become blood glucose, the brain's preferred fuel for high-effort situations. The brain can run on partially broken down fats (called *ketones*) during a low-carb diet, but thought processes will never be consistently as strong compared to ticking by on glucose from carbs.

THE GOVERNOR DECIDES

Recent research has shown in endurance athletes, even the *perception* of carbs in the mouth can affect how fast you're likely to run. This is called the **Central Governor Theory**. If the brain senses you're going to fuel it generously, it responds by giving you a general mojo to *go for it*. This is likely to be proven in strength athletes soon. High energy levels mean you will get better numbers in your workouts - more reps, sets and poundages - thereby stimulating more muscle growth. I'll repeat the earlier statement as a final reminder:

We need carbs to get swole.

******

So what's left if we've ditched percentages, grams and even calories? There is a very sensible approach, and it arrives in two servings. It relates to why most of us like carbs in the first place.

NUTRIENTS

The number one reason humans seek carbs is because they come packaged *with* nutrients. This is why species with a poor sense of taste and no access to quality food, have to eat *lots*. A panda is a good example, needing 90 pounds (40kg) of bamboo *a day* to reach minimum nutrient levels.

What nutrients do humans seek? We're not talking about energy yet (calories), we're talking nutrients. They are: vitamins, minerals, and what we call *phytonutrients* or *phytochemicals*. "Phyto" means from plants. There could be hundreds, or possibly thousands of nutrients that make humans *thrive*. Everything with a strong color contains a benefit, with plant pigments protecting various aspects of our health. The nice sweet or savory tastes that natural food comes with is Mother Nature's bribe, her "dinner's ready" call to get us to the table.

In addition to phytonutrients, we need fiber, the non-digestible, non-nutrient part of our food. This scrubs out our insides, and improves the digestive process. It can also help keep blood sugar more stable, as fiber slows the *early* part of digestion, where foods release their goodies into the blood. Think of fiber as nature's *Mobil 1*, keeping our "engine" well maintained. We also get some water from food.

Let's head back to the zoo to visit our panda friend, who's stuck on a diet of *bamboo*. Bamboo is low in nutrients. Very. As such, panda has to eat lots (no wonder they never have time to breed). When humans eat the opposite of bamboo, i.e. highly nutritious food - or what geeks call **high nutrient density** - we eat slightly less overall. That's a fat-loss "secret" in a sentence. Eat high nutrient density foods, and you'll lose your gut *fast*. You'll consume less energy and more fiber (which physically makes eating difficult). For us, this has health positives, and some swole negatives, which we'll cover in a bit. Before we do that, let's consider other reasons we instinctively thrive on carbs.

ENERGY

It's plain old calories. Humans eat carbs as they provide an easy fuel. All foods eventually convert to the universal energy molecule, ATP (adenosine triphosphate). Carbs have the easiest commute to becoming ATP, which is handy as it powers our entire machine. I don't just mean muscle, I mean processes at the cellular level and *throughout* the entire body. Our heart, other organs, immune system, hormone system, nervous system, repair system, thoughts, and even digestion itself, *all* need ATP. I am concerned with those, but our biggest goal is fueling the artificial process known as **muscular hypertrophy**, i.e. getting swole. Because you train (and train harder than split-system saps), you need lots of ATP. Full-body workouts "stress" the entire system, and recovery forces your "factory" into full-tilt production, 24/7. The factory works smoothest with a decent flow of ATP. It's that simple.

Right, you have the reasons behind carb effectiveness, and why we naturally go for them. We need to combine everything into a workable swole strategy. I'm going to sneak in a percentage (technically, a ratio), but it's so easy you won't mind. Importantly, you'll love its results.

THE HALF AND HALF PRINCIPLE

Mentally, you just need to do **one** deceptively simple thing for mealtime carbs.

You need to fill *half* your plate, or whatever you put food on, with starchy carbs. Examples of these are:

- Rice (white, brown, wholemeal)
- Potatoes (new, sweet, jacket, baked, roasted)
- Breads (wholemeal, avoid white)
- Pasta (white, wholemeal)
- Noodles (egg, non-egg)
- Porridge (oats / oatmeal)

Add your favorite dressing or sauce to ensure stickability. And on the other half, you add fruits or vegetables. I won't list those, as the list is endless. Mixing colors is always the smartest strategy. How *much* of each?

If you pick natural foods (things *without* long labels, and things *with* a short expiry date), simply eat using appetite.

So what's the deal with this simple system, and, where's the protein and fat? Well, we need <u>*at least* half of the plate filled with starchy carbs</u>, as eating them will allow you to get enough *easily* converted energy for ATP. Remember, ATP powers your workouts, but also your recovery from them. And, you want <u>*at most* half of the plate filled with fruit or veg</u>. Why at most?

Because if you went crazy on them, their superior nutrient density, fiber and water content would mean you eat less energy overall. Not ideal, as you're not an Average Joe. You're a full-body beast!

There will be days you crave a *whole* plate of starchy carbs. If that happens, go for it. Don't do it all the time, as even *Super Swolers* benefit from more phytonutrients. I doubt that you'd ever want to do the reverse, i.e. live off a whole plate of fruit and veg, but if you do, do that just as rarely, at least while on the program.

"But what about the protein?" you're still screaming. Well, I don't mention protein *or* fat because that complicates and confuses. Protein foods tend to come without many carbs, so you can regard them as a separate part of meals, i.e. **just focus on hitting your daily protein target**. As for fat, don't *seek* it, with the exception of some extra virgin olive oil, and maybe the odd bit of omega 3. Let's simplify.

Protein is about hitting your daily grams, and fat takes care of itself. To gauge carbs, just fill at least half of your plate with starchy carbs you enjoy, and fruit and veg to make up the rest. You don't literally have to put everything *on* a plate, but at least use a "virtual" plate to guide you.

Finally, eat according to appetite.

This may sound like a simplistic system, and it is. It also works. Give it a try and you'll discover to your delight, it's really do-able. Why do I have faith in this system? Apart from the fact it works, there's an extra reason, and one that everyone has access to.

THE BODY FAT BUFFER

We all have an in-built mechanism to ensure our success. That mechanism is called *body fat*. Our chubby bits represent nature's greatest lifesaver, or even banker. Body fat contains about 3500 calories per pound (it varies as people vary in *their* fat's water content). Even in the leanest folk, there is spare pudge. With such calorie density, body fat is always there to pick up the pieces if you don't consume enough energy (calories). **It's literally why we have it**.

And of course, when your calculations are a bit out, and you eat too much, we store some of that excess away. Body fat isn't our first choice fuel, but it's the perfect background partner to balance inaccuracies in our daily carb selection and appetite. Put simply, **body fat is your autopilot, taking the controls when necessary**. If you train consistently, eat enough protein, and fill half your plate with quality starchy carbs, you will be perfectly placed to fuel your muscle growth. And you'll overeat rarely.

This system really does work. Give it a few days and make it a habit. I doubt you'll go back to anything else.

Before we head off, it's worth discussing a common fear about carbs, even amongst guys who aren't generally *that* scared of them.

NIGHT TIME TERRORS

Many people - *most* - seem to believe that carbs eaten at night make you fat.

This idea originally came from low-carb dieters, who obsessed about eating all their carbs by a certain cut-off point on the clock.

For example, "eat all your carbs by 6pm". This technique was successful in increasing weight loss, mainly because when you cut *anything* off early, you have a lot less of *everything*. Annoyingly, the idea caught on, and people now associate late-night carbs with "there tomorrow" fat.

Extensive research, including meta-analyses (studies of *all* the studies), show that carb timing tends to *not* make much difference to body fat. Obviously we are interested in muscle, but the point's still interesting. The point being, your body is smarter than just monitoring what you do by the clock, and even what you do according to the light/dark cycle. **You must not be afraid of eating carbs, regardless of what the clock says**. You can have them in every meal if you wish.

Humans are social creatures, and your success with *Super Swole* is largely connected with your ability to make it part of your life, or at least 6 weeks of it. Night happens to be the time humans meet, and laying down rules about carb timing goes against how we roll. From a physiological perspective, newer research reveals we may even be *designed* to eat more carbs at night. Carbs boost dopamine, the feel-good brain chemical, and then serotonin, another neurotransmitter. These stimulate our *para-sympathetic nervous system*. This chills us out, making us feel calm and **happy**. Happy is in bold for a reason; it's a human end goal. The opposite system - the *sympathetic nervous system* - is dominant during the day. It charges us up, and makes us run around to get stuff done. It's *power by adrenaline*. Before we get too scientifically deep, just take this one message home:

We are programmed to enjoy food at night, including carbs, so don't be afraid of them at any of your 4 meals; pick foods you *enjoy*, which also happen to have some health benefits.

So, that's carbs. Forget grams, percentages, and ratios between your other macros. Fill at least half your plate with starchy carbs, and whatever's left with fruit or veg. Go for quality, taste, and fill your boots.

BRO VS PRO

bro

× just eat tons of carbs
× don't eat carbs man, go paleo
× it's all about calories dude

pro

✓ carbs efficiently boost ATP, the best fuel for *Super Swole*
✓ you don't need to count grams or daily carb proportions
✓ fill at least half your plate with starchy carbs; add fruit & veg

CREATINE

A few chapters back, I said there were 5 macronutrients, 3 of which - protein, fat and carbs - we've discussed. The other two are easy. For fiber, just eat enough good carbs, including fruit and veg, and then you're all set. And for water, just obey your thirst. Despite people saying otherwise, thirst is a good hydration indicator. Instead, we'll investigate two other diet-related components. In terms of getting swole, I'm almost tempted to call them macros. They are *whey protein* and *creatine*. If you can tolerate these, they'll accelerate your progress. This chapter is about creatine.

Creatine is one of two supplements (the other being protein) that have stood the test of time. In 1992, a trio of highly successful British Olympic athletes - two gold medalists and a world record holder* - openly mentioned their use of it, and the athletic media got hooked. I talked to the leading British high jumper at the time, who said he *didn't* take it because it made him "too powerful"! He suggested that the extra "bounce" put him at a greater risk of injury. In short, creatine had a buzz about it, because it actually seemed *to do something*.

Despite the buzz, it wasn't until the mid 1990s that supplement company *EAS* managed to produce something for the public. When they released their first creatine product, *Phosphagen*, it flew off the shelves. Ever since, companies have been clucking for a piece of the market.

The truth is, creatine was actually discovered 160 years before the Olympic Brits got their hands on it. In 1832, a French chemist extracted some from muscle, and named it *creatine*, the Greek word for *flesh*.

THE THREE AMINOS

Technically, creatine is a peptide protein. That's a structure made of a few amino acids joined together. Creatine is made of three aminos: *arginine*, *glycine* and *methionine*. These are combined in your liver to make creatine, which then gets sent around. Over 90% is in your muscle, with some left over for your brain, eyes, blood, and central nervous system.

YOU ARE WHAT YOU EAT

If you eat meat, you're literally eating the dead muscles of animals. When they're killed, their muscles contain creatine. If you eat *their* muscles, you eat *their* creatine. Put simply, **if you eat meat, you're already using a creatine supplement**. In addition to getting creatine from meat, your liver makes between 1 and 2 grams daily. The exact figure is difficult to measure. We know we definitely produce some, because vegetarians and vegans don't have creatine *in their diet* and yet they still generate the same power as carnivores. Having said that, when vegetarians or vegans take a creatine supplement, their levels rise dramatically, with research showing they get the biggest benefit (good karma perhaps). Meat eaters get benefits too, but slightly less. It depends on how "topped up" the muscles already are. So, you're dosed up on creatine history, and you know what it is, but you're desperate to ask, "does it do anything?'. Here we go.

THE BENEFITS OF CREATINE

There are benefits. Some of them are hype, while others are actually not talked about despite being important.

Because there's *so* much research on creatine, and so much written in broscience, it's hard to make sense of it all. Plus of course, whenever big business is involved, finding the truth becomes difficult. Let's tackle the questions I hear all the time.

WILL IT MAKE ME SPRINT FASTER?

No. Usain Bolt won't panic just because you find a cheap deal on monohydrate. But if you had to do 10 sprints in 10 minutes, taking creatine would help you recover quicker *between* runs, giving you faster *average* times over the whole session. If you were to consistently do *that*, it's possible that creatine would *indirectly* make you faster. Multiple sets in the gym are similar to multiple sprints.

WILL IT MAKE ME STRONGER?

Possibly. Results are mixed. The problem is, strength is affected by endless factors. Food, sleep, having the right training program, how happy you are, and how focused you are *that* day. This makes studying the link with strength almost impossible.

Ask guys at the gym if it makes them stronger, and you'll probably get varied answers. Some will swear by it, others will say it's junk. And a few might admit to taking it without feeling anything (they won't stop for fear of giving away an edge).

In theory, creatine could make you stronger simply because it draws more water into the muscle. **A muscle that's fully hydrated is stronger than a dehydrated muscle**. Why? Because muscle fibers line up better and slide over each other for a more efficient contraction. Having enough liquid in your diet generally takes care of this, but creatine tends to increase muscle water content slightly above that of a non-user.

The extra water weight affects people differently. Some gain 5 to 7 pounds within a week and maintain it for as long as they're "on". Others gain the same and then gradually lose it. And finally, others don't notice *any* change in weight. We aren't sure why that happens. Scientists call these people *non-responders*. They assume if someone's weight doesn't change, and if they can't shift more weight in the gym, they're not responding. We'll see later on, that this isn't necessarily true.

A true non-responder is someone whose *measured* levels of *muscle* creatine doesn't change. How are levels measured? It's called a **muscle biopsy**. This involves a local anesthetic jab, and then a sliver of muscle being taken via a large needle. That's then analyzed with chemicals and microscope. True creatine non-responders are rare. If you work out, your muscles are above average in terms of how they absorb *any* nutrient or chemical. Literally, one decent workout takes the surface of worked muscles from being like normal paper to being like blotting paper (or toilet paper, if you've no idea what blotting paper is). This enhancement lasts just about 24 hours by the way, perhaps a hint from Mother Nature to encourage daily activity.

As for creatine increasing your strength directly, it's unlikely. Its main job in the body is to help out its friend, ATP (adenosine triphosphate). ATP is an energy molecule - *a fuel source* - used in multiple activities from blinking to sprinting, to the general powering of all our cells. In fact ATP helps any kind of *-ing* you can think of. Yep, even that.

But even though ATP is the powerhouse in strength training, it runs out of steam after about 4 or 5 reps. That's roughly the same as 5 or 6 seconds of all-out effort. Elite 100-meter sprinters get faster from when the gun bangs - to about 60 meters - i.e. until 6 seconds on the clock. At this point, their ATP runs flat, and then the winner is the athlete who *slows down the least*. In terms of hitting weights, after about 5 to 6 reps, creatine could help you to pump out a few more. These extra reps themselves could stimulate more muscle growth. You have to train *hard* to get this as a benefit.

So far, it probably sounds like creatine doesn't deserve all this space, so why even mention it? Because it has one less talked about effect, and it's the most important.

SATELLITE CELL ACTIVATION

Okay, it might sound like a geek subtitle, but it's crucial. Modern sport science has discovered that at least some muscle growth is triggered by activating small cells that hang around regular muscle cells. They're called **satellite cells**. Normally, they just sit there, almost asleep. With mechanical tension, i.e. lifting weight, they spring into action. It all makes sense really. If you repeatedly work your muscles hard, the body adapts by making your muscles bigger and stronger. The satellite cells join with regular muscle cells, making them swell up. Super Swole! This could happen as satellite cells donate their *nucleus*, that being the DNA and "hard drive" containing part of the cell. By satellite cells donating their "brain", the new double-brained muscle cells increase protein production and *ta-da*, your muscles get bigger.

There is research that suggests even diet can activate these little helpers. It's at an early stage, and so I can't officially push it here. But I can say, studies show creatine supplements help activate *extra* satellite cell activity. This is why studies tend to find creatine users grow faster than non-users. When you combine creatine, heavy training and a good diet, the effect is powerful. By activating *lots* of satellite cells, you are giving your muscles the greatest statistical chance to grow. In a short period of time, e.g. during a 7 day study, it's not always easy to spot this. But give it 6 weeks and beyond, and you'll start to get extra benefits.

So, having turned it around and put creatine in everyone's good books, is there anything else to consider. Of course.

THE DANGERS OF A WHITE POWDER

Do they exist? Yes. Most people will throw down broscience and copy what they've heard elsewhere:

- creatine is 100% safe
- you can take it forever without problems
- only people with kidney problems shouldn't take it

All proteins - and creatine *is* a protein peptide - are processed by various parts of the body, especially the kidneys. With a high intake of dietary protein, kidneys have to work hard anyway. And extra creatine *could* increase their "stress" even more. Would you know about it? If you're young, you probably wouldn't notice. But, that doesn't mean it's "safe". All the broscientists who claim it's entirely safe, state this without *ever* having had a blood test themselves.

Apart from this effect on the kidneys, what else can creatine do? At least one study shows that regular supplementation with creatine can raise **dihydrotestosterone** (by 40%).

This cousin of testosterone can, if your genes are programmed for it, increase male pattern baldness, and *possibly* enlarge the prostate. The idea that creatine, a protein peptide, could somehow affect hormones is not well known. Our hormones are *very* finely balanced, and if you knock one out of sync, there's a chance that you could knock the whole system out. I'm not saying creatine does this, because honestly, I don't know. No one does yet. I'm just saying, it *could*.

Smaller potential problems are stomach upsets, and extra toilet visits. These two problems generally *only* happen if you load creatine, something not strictly necessary (we'll chat about it in a bit). Although there have been "long-term" safety studies (e.g. 5 years), no research is 100% perfect.

We can only measure what we actually look for, and who knows if there's something else we haven't even thought of.

PROOF

Almost all the decent studies on creatine, have used a form called **creatine monohydrate**. This is the only form you should bother buying. Why can I say that with certainty? Because monohydrate *is* very well absorbed - almost 100% - which is unusual for any substance. And once your muscles are topped up with creatine, <u>any form of it</u> - no matter how fancy - <u>cannot push muscle levels even higher</u>.

Muscles *full* of creatine, that's about 25% more than Average Joe, are like a sponge *full* of water. Once your muscles are fully saturated, no matter what you chuck at them (i.e. different types of creatine), they can't take any more. It just spills over. Fine if you're a sponge over a sink, not so fine if that sink is *your* kidneys.

Creatine monohydrate is the form most widely produced, and that means it's the cheapest. The only thing I encourage is for you to buy from a big company. A well-known business will want to protect its reputation, and this means they'll take better care of what they sell. Most of them don't actually *make* creatine (they buy it from wholesalers), but they will test batches to make sure it's safe for their customers.

Impure creatine has been found to contain toxic metals, and once in the body, metals rarely leave.

Although I cannot recommend brands in general, a German producer makes a type of high quality creatine that's routinely tested for impurities.

It's called *Creapure*, and it's the same type used in most research. All the good supplement brands will offer a product sourced from it. For a few pennies extra, it's worth it.

HOW MUCH?

As mentioned earlier, it's not necessary to "load" creatine. Taking 20 grams in a day, for *one* day, is the limit of sensible *fast* loading. Studies show that by day 2, you're peeing out most of the rest. A smart amount is:

- take 5 to 6 grams on training days after training
- take *half* that on non-training days with a meal

Why take it *after* training? Because training makes your muscle tissue surfaces more absorbent for 1 to 2 hours. The entire goal of creatine supplementation is to build up muscle levels to their maximum. Actually, to about 25% over what's considered "normal". And then, to keep it there. It's this super saturation that stimulates satellite cells to boost protein synthesis (muscle growth). Taking creatine post-workout is optimal. At this time, you'll be taking in some post-workout nutrients, hopefully a protein shake and some carbs. The carbs raise insulin, a hormone that takes nutrients from the blood and helps escort them into muscle cells. Even a large dose of protein can boost insulin. All of this helps "pull" creatine into the muscle. More about the post-workout shake later.

On non-training days, taking roughly 3 grams will keep your levels from dropping. Although it's not essential to combine it with food, taking this small dose with a meal will give you better odds at absorbing *all* of it. Within 14 to 21 days of taking small amounts of creatine, your muscle levels will be brimming over.

GETTING OFF YOUR CYCLE

A real controversy is whether to cycle creatine. That is, to take it for a bit, and get off it for a bit. The original recommendations were to cycle. The idea was to use creatine for 8 weeks, and come off it for 4, then start again. Modern research has found that after 4 weeks of stopping, levels aren't completely down to those before taking it. So, cycling off for 4 weeks isn't enough for a proper rest. Based on the stats, it's likely that 6 to 8 weeks are necessary to hit "normal" again. But what about the longer-term new research that shows people can take creatine continuously for years? The broscience of today keeps quoting this, and saying smugly that creatine is perfectly fine for constant use. I beg to differ.

First of all, we have only researched *some* variables in these studies. As mentioned earlier, there could be things we should look for, but we don't even know *what* those things are. Secondly, just because studies show no "damaging" effects, it doesn't mean the body won't benefit from a complete rest. And finally, there's a definite psychological boost from having a clean-out break, and then going back "on". So, I'd still cycle creatine, despite the current trend. Use it for up to 8 weeks, and then come off for 8 weeks.

Creatine may be naturally produced, but natural doesn't mean harmless. There are "natural" frogs in the Amazon rainforest which are deadlier than our best *man-made* poison! The bottom line: we just don't know. If creatine is something you can tolerate, use it sensibly, make great gains, and respect it by cycling.

*The three British athletes who made creatine popular were: Linford Christie, 1992 Olympic Gold Medalist in the 100m; Sally Gunnell, 1992 Olympic Gold Medalist and World Record holder in the 400m Hurdles; Colin Jackson, 110m Hurdles World Record holder.

BRO VS PRO

bro

- ✗ creatine does nothing / everything
- ✗ creatine just blows you up with water
- ✗ creatine will make you stronger / faster in a week

pro

- ✓ creatine enhances muscle growth at the cellular level
- ✓ don't load; take 5-6g on training days, 3g at other times
- ✓ use creatine for 8 weeks max, and then give it 8 weeks off

WHEY PROTEIN

Along with creatine, protein powders have been the biggest success in sports nutrition. In fact they're bigger than creatine, as even the mainstream public use them. Although mentioned by ancient Greek physician *Hippocrates*, you have to fast forward to 18th century Britain for records of people drinking "whey". And the product we now recognize didn't land until '93, when legendary steroid guru *Dan Duchaine* launched *Designer Whey*.

But what is it? It's one half of the proteins in milk. Well, it's 20% in real terms, with the other 80% being *casein*. Casein is a slow released protein, which becomes a thick gel in the stomach, taking 7 hours to digest. Whey on the other hand, raises blood levels of aminos within 20 minutes - peaks in 1 hour - and is out of your system in 3. Mother's milk (human mothers) is about 60% whey, and 40% casein.

MILKING THE ACCURACY

A *closer* look at mother's milk stats (oh yes, I did this) reveals something interesting. When a baby is born and the mother *starts* breast-feeding, her milk is 80% whey and 20% casein. That's 80% fast proteins and 20% slow release. Around 6 months later when the baby is nearly *finished* breast-feeding, it's a 50:50 split. Did Mother Nature realize that a baby's early growth needs faster protein? It seems so. And that's exactly why modern day whey supplements make great post-workout proteins. Before you ask, stealing mother's milk is probably a crime. And definitely awkward. I'll continue.

The post-workout "window" of opportunity, roughly lasting for 1 to 2 hours, is useful for those wanting to **maximize** muscle mass.

Again, broscience will tell you that this time isn't important, and that as long as you get enough protein *at some point*, you'll be fine. I'm sorry guys, but that just isn't true. In beginners, it's *partially* true. Their bodies suck up nutrients 'round the clock. And those same beginners tend not to train with much intensity (they haven't learned how to). In short, they're not stimulating that much growth.

Also, in the first few weeks of a program, the body tends to get stronger *without* getting much bigger. This happens because the entire nervous system gets better wiring. Your body literally grows more connections, allowing more electrical power to fire-up muscle. This allows the body to sneakily cope with the "stress" *without* needing to build calorie-hungry muscle. This is why many studies - which use complete beginners - don't show much difference in terms of protein timing.

Earlier research on protein absorption revealed another clue. In experienced lifters, they noticed a more *efficient* use of protein. That is, compared to newer lifters, they absorbed more and wasted less. The researchers did these studies to see how much protein was needed *in general*. In doing them, they created a big clue about protein timing:

The more experienced you are, and the harder you train, the <u>faster</u> your body needs protein.

The window of opportunity always exists, but it gets much smaller.

So bros, continue mocking those with a shaker in the locker room if you like, but they're actually doing the smart thing: getting aminos in *fast*.

THE SECRET WHEY

The reason whey is generally powerful, apart from its speed, is its *amino acid content*. Over half of its protein is **essential**, i.e. the amino acids we humans specifically need to grow. Of those, whey also contains high amounts of Branch Chain Amino Acids (BCAAs). These are uniquely structured amino acids (*leucine*, *isoleucine* and *valine*) that contribute to endurance and growth. Whey is particularly high in **leucine**, an amino acid now understood to trigger the entire muscle-building cascade. As whey protein *is* mainly protein, it also becomes useful when dieting. High levels of aminos, particularly BCAAs, help prevent muscle loss on low-calorie diets. Dieting is beyond this book, but it's useful to be aware of this quality.

WHAT WHEY SHOULD I GO?

There are many types of whey, all with fancy sounding names. The basic types are:

- concentrate
- isolate
- hydrolysate

Concentrate is the cheapest form, and in an average of 100 grams of dry powder, it has about 80 grams of actual protein. The rest contains some fat, and a sugar called *lactose*, also known as milk sugar.

Lactose is the one problem that whey presents in some people. Many adult humans don't have a problem, but some do, especially black, Asian and southern Europeans.

Certain gene holders tend to get stomach rumbles if they have too much lactose. They are *lactose intolerant*. This means not having enough of the enzyme *lactase*, a chemical needed to breakdown lact-*ose* before it gets too far down the pipe. As a result, it "cooks" up inside them (breaks down incompletely), causing gas or worse (you'll see a sprint for the toilet).

If this is you, you're better off getting whey **isolate**. This has more protein per 100 grams (from 90 to almost 100), and crucially, almost no lactose. The protein itself isn't any better than what's in concentrate, but the lactose content is lower. Of course you have to pay for this, and whey isolate is quite a bit more expensive than concentrate. As always, the best advice is to really pick your parents!

Finally, there's **hydrolysate**. This is whey protein that's already been pre-digested. Sounds disgusting I know. Chemicals are used to chop up some of the bonds - or linkages - between parts of the whey. This makes it even faster to absorb. While this sounds cool, I don't recommend you buy this type. Firstly, it's not necessary, as concentrate and isolate are already the fastest proteins on the planet. And secondly, breaking up the bonds *could* make the protein less healthy. Whey is known for its immune boosting properties, something that's useful after a workout (when immunity naturally dips). Whey boosts immunity because it contains an amino acid called **cysteine**. Once inside you, your body converts this to an antioxidant called **glutathione**. This is your body's natural, self-made multi vitamin. Well it's not strictly a vitamin or a mineral, but a protector of your body. This immune boosting quality makes whey an ideal protein for general use. Staying sick means staying out of the gym. Let's do a quick recap.

Whey protein is a valuable supplement. It's not essential for all of your daily protein, but used after workouts, it's particularly effective.

BRO VS PRO

bro

- ✕ all whey is the same
- ✕ just take what I take
- ✕ whey is like steroids

pro

- ✓ whey is useful for post-workout nutrition
- ✓ whey has high levels of essential amino acids & BCAAs
- ✓ concentrate works for most, while some could need an isolate

THE POST-WORKOUT SHAKE

So, the time has come to discuss the most important of your 4 daily meals (sorry Mr Breakfast). And, it's probably the most important thing you need to get right other than training itself. You're already dosed up on macros, and you know quite a bit about whey and creatine, so let's put it all together. Say hello to my little friend: the **post-workout shake**.

Your post-workout shake needs at least one component. To be better than most brews, it needs two. And ideally, it needs a third. Put another way:

1 component   **good**
2 components   **even better**
3 components   **look at my arms baby!**

COMPONENT #1 = PROTEIN

Consume liquid protein within 15 and 30 minutes after working out. This must contain at least 20 grams of protein, and ideally, 40.

By now, I've probably driven you mad by repeating things over and over. But it's necessary, especially today when legions of broscientists spout convincing arguments about why you shouldn't be seen with a shaker in public. They may even show you their great body for proof. While that's nice for them, it *doesn't* mean they got there as quickly as they could have.

Liquid protein is the vital first bit of your post-workout (abbreviated to: PWO) shake. The amount, 20 to 40 grams, is critical too. Anything less than 20 grams puts you at risk. Studies which conclude 20 grams is the *maximum* necessary, often use untrained subjects who just hit a few sets of leg extensions. This is not the typical *Super Swole* user. Full-body workouts are great, but they're tough, and it's likely that close to the whole 40 grams of post-workout protein will come in handy. In guys who are 40 years old or older, 40 grams of protein has already showed better results than 20 grams. Their protein absorption is a little less efficient than younger guys, at least in the beginning. If you are on a mission to get swole, I would head towards 40 grams of protein whatever your birth certificate says. Anything more than 40 grams though, has not been demonstrated to have any benefits (in any group).

Aim for 40 grams of protein.

What about the source? It is important. Recent research has discovered one particular amino acid as having more power than the rest.

Leucine.

We mentioned this briefly as one of the 8 **Essential Amino Acids** (EAAs). For some reason, leucine triggers a gene and protein complex in the body called **mTOR**. I'm going to give you short paragraphs to take this in. Stay calm!

Right.

mTOR, also known as, wait for it - **mechanistic target of rapamycin** - or even better - **mammalian target of rapamycin** - are genes and proteins which trigger growth, including muscle growth.

Leucine triggers mTOR, and mTOR makes muscles grow.

Exercise *also* triggers mTOR, but in combination with a leucine-rich protein, the effect is boosted massively. Another reason why you want to eat soon after training, as mTOR gradually goes down after. Most protein foods contain leucine (but undeniably, one has more than most). Here's the liquid list, in order of most to least:

- Whey protein
- Soy protein (isolate)
- Milk (skim)
- Beef protein (isolate)

Now it's worth remembering that leucine might not be the *only* trigger of mTOR, but it's the one we know about now. All of the proteins in the list contain a general mix of proteins, including enough of all the essential amino acids. Here's the quick comparison of these fantastic four.

WHEY

It's the ultimate party guest: fast in, fast out, and it mixes well. It can also have its taste easily disguised, and doesn't cost much.

Whey concentrate is for those who can tolerate *lactose* (milk sugar), and whey isolate is for those who can't. Whey also has immune boosting properties. It's easy to get up to 40 grams of protein from whey, with around 50 grams (less than two ounces) of actual powder needed. If you go for whey, just mix it with water to maintain its speed. Milk will slow it down a bit.

If you can take whey, make it your #1 PWO choice.

SOY PROTEIN (ISOLATE)

It's a relatively fast protein, but not as fast as whey. The leucine content is good. There are some concerns over its estrogen-like qualities, but this has <u>not</u> been shown in good research. An isolate of soy is less common than whey, and more expensive generally. If you cannot get on with whey, it's a useful alternative. Bear in mind, undigested soy proteins can cause gas in some people. Taste wise, it's faint and hard to mask, with companies using apple sugar or a natural sweetener. Both are fine for post-workout. Soy isolate is similar to whey, in that you don't need much powder to get lots of actual protein.

If you are anti animal foods, or don't get on with whey, soy isolate is a good alternative.

MILK (SKIM)

Good old milk protein has been around since Arnold's time (even though he cheekily once said "no skim milk, milk is for babies"). The protein content is solid across all the aminos, plus of course, cow's milk is 20% whey.

The remaining 80% is casein, a traditionally "slow" protein. In real life studies, skim milk seems to be absorbed faster post-workout. Casein in cheese and yogurt is slower, but in a liquid form and *without* fat, skim milk gets in at an acceptable speed.

If you're on a budget, it's a no-brainer. Go organic if you can. Remember, to get 20 grams of protein, you'll need about half a quart / 500 mls, and to get 40, double that. It is possible. The benefit of all this liquid is that you'll please your kidneys. The downside: you'll need to be near a toilet 60 minutes later.

Incidentally, if you are going with milk, read on later, as adding carbs post-workout is useful. In which case, you can be naughty with milk, and have some with *sugar*...

BEEF PROTEIN

The idea of *cow-in-liquid* isn't that appetizing (especially not for the cow). A relatively new addition to protein powders, beef protein isolate contains a decent amount of leucine, but only just. It's slower than whey also. Mainly, the benefit of beef is for those who cannot tolerate whey and don't like soy or milk. There may be traces of creatine in beef protein, but it would be a stretch to call it a creatine supplement.

Taste wise, well, what can I say. It's not everyone's cup of tea. Or beef. Perhaps the closest estimate is that it's like a beef stock. If you cannot get on with any of the first three proteins, maybe try some. It's quite dense, so you won't need much powder.

If you get 40 grams *of protein* from any of these guys, you should be getting enough leucine. **Roughly 2 to 3 grams** is all you need to trigger mTOR. Some protein powders *add* leucine. You will pay more for this, and it's not necessary.

In fact, it could be less useful, as nature tends to *never* "spike" its proteins in the same way. Do not buy or use leucine supplements. Okay, time to move onto the next thing you need.

COMPONENT #2 = CREATINE

We've had a whole section on this stuff, so hopefully you're convinced. Remember, **creatine stimulates satellite cells**, small helper cells who donate themselves to muscle cells, accelerating growth. Research has shown a combination of whey and creatine to be very powerful. Perhaps other proteins would combine with creatine well also, but they've rarely been researched. Try and get *Creapure* sourced creatine monohydrate. Lots of companies use it now.

Get 5 to 6 grams of creatine monohydrate in your post-workout shake.

I suggest you mix your creatine **separately** from your protein (and carbs). Why? No matter what form you buy - including *micronized* - it will sink to the bottom of your shaker. Fast. 5 to 6 grams is not much powder at all, and there is a possibility that you will leave most of your creatine at the bottom of your shaker if you don't properly mix and gulp.

The simplest and most effective way to deliver creatine, is in a plain water bottle. That way you can *see it* clearly, and add a bit more water if you've left any at the bottom. Creatine has no taste, but it does have a texture. Like very fine sand. It's not horrible. Just think you're having fun at the beach.

******

The final piece of the post-workout puzzle is below, and broscientists, get ready to be angry.

COMPONENT #3 = CARBS

Okay, carbs seem to have lost their friends these days, especially in gym circles. In the 70s, carbs were the *only* things recommended by sport scientists. Then in the 80s and 90s, they were recommended with protein. Finally, in the naughties and 10s they started disappearing from recommendations. Why? Because carbs are the new villains accused of making the world fat. While this is true in *some* ways, it's not strictly true. My analogy is the speed of a car. Sometimes, driving fast is dangerous. And other times, like on a freeway, it's appropriate. Carbs and cars, not too different. Fast carbs have limited use in an Average Joe's diet. Yet again, I have to remind you, you're not him.

After a workout, especially a full-body workout, you'll have used up lots of internally stored muscle carbs, aka *glycogen*. Given a normal diet, these stores will slowly top-up. I cannot deny that. But your focus, your obsession, is not about gently gliding along with normal processes. Because if you do, your gains will suffer. I can hear the broscientists getting angry in the wings.

Carbs, protein and creatine definitely have a *synergistic* effect. That is, they're like 1+1+1 = 5. **Carbs boost insulin**, the body's main storage hormone. Although protein and creatine can get into muscle cells without insulin, carbs speed up the process dramatically. Why is this important?

Your body's muscle protein is usually in one of two states:

MPB (muscle protein breakdown)
MPS (muscle protein synthesis)

It's the balance between these two which determines whether your muscles get bigger or smaller. Exercise, with weights especially, tends to increase muscle protein breakdown. Adding protein to your shake will increase muscle protein synthesis. To let protein maximize this job, carbs really help balance the other side of the equation:

Carbs, probably through boosting insulin, reduce muscle protein breakdown.

This is the double whammy you want. Get protein to increase building, and get carbs to stop the bulldozing. Rome wasn't built in a day, but it would have been built quicker on creatine, protein *and* carbs.

Carbs, as mentioned, also increase the speed at which creatine gets into muscles. Although I would hope your creatine levels are already being kept high, it's possible that shoveling more creatine post-workout *triggers* satellite cell activation *in-the-moment*, boosting how fast your muscles grow in the hours just after training.

Another lesser-known thing about carbs, is that they stop the build up of **AMPK**. Okay, I have to give you its full name:

5' adenosine monophosphate-activated protein kinase

It's an enzyme which increases fat burning, stops your liver making cholesterol, and it opposes our post-workout friend, mTOR.

While fat burning is nice, it's not appropriate if you're trying to get swole in a hurry. And while dropping cholesterol might be healthy for life overall, it's not great if you're trying to build mass. Cholesterol is actually the first material to make testosterone, and it's also the carrier that transports it around your body.

The last thing you want to do is take away testosterone's ride in the hours after you workout.

Simply put, post-workout carbs are anabolic.

They have too many benefits to ignore for those with swole dreams. How much is useful? Now of course we all vary in size, including muscle tissue, but I can hear you screaming for a recommendation. Here it is:

Get 40 to 60 grams of liquid carbs in your post-workout shake.

I have given you a 20-gram range, because that's practical, depending on where you get your carbs. Ideally, you go liquid. You should be sold on post-workout liquids by now.

If you choose whey or beef for your protein, you will be getting little carbs (less than 10 grams for sure). If you choose soy, it all depends on the brand. Some are like whey or beef (i.e. low carb). Others are heavily sweetened with sugars, and therefore might solve your carb problem without you trying.

Interestingly, if you opt for milk, there will be carbs of plenty (lactose). This itself should be enough, but you *may* be able to get away with a slightly sweetened version, i.e. chocolate or strawberry milk. Result!

Whatever the case, if you are adding carbs, don't worry about the source too much. In post-workout mode, your body will scoop them up regardless of their glycemic index (the speed at which they leak carbs into the blood).

FAST AND FURIOUS

Glucose powder - known as **dextrose** - is cheap, and quite palatable. It gets into the system fast, and it doesn't generally cause bloat. Don't go for any other special carb supplements, as they cannot do much beyond plain old dextrose.

Fruit juice is not recommended. *Some* fruit juices contain a slightly high concentration of *fructose* (fruit sugar), and this can reduce the way insulin works. That would potentially mean less protein and less creatine getting into your muscles. For the record, fructose in *whole* fruits seems <u>not</u> to damage how insulin works. Still, most fruit is a bit slow for our purposes.

A **commercial sports drink**, as in one bought from a regular store, is perfect. Plus, it's a nice treat after a hard session. Remember, you need between **40 and 60 grams of carbs**. Some sports drinks are much lower as they're designed to be drunk *during* your workout. That's a useful reminder:

Do not drink anything other than plain water during your workout.

Other drinks during your workout aren't necessary, and can tempt you to have poorer pre-workout meals. You begin to *rely* on their sugary boost for maintaining your workout intensity. Not good. Plus they damage your teeth, and may reduce the boost of having carbs, proteins and creatine *after* your workout.

If you can't find dextrose (glucose) or a sugary sports drink you enjoy, then it would still be better for you to have *something*. Although liquids are preferred, two bananas, or two pieces of other fruits will make do.

Okay, you're probably getting tired now, so here's a sum up of what to do post-workout:

1) Consume a liquid protein within 15 and 30 minutes after working out. This must contain at least 20 grams of protein, and ideally, 40 grams. Choose whey, soy isolate, skim milk or beef isolate.

2) Get 5 to 6 grams of creatine monohydrate in your post-workout shake. Try and find a brand with *Creapure*, and mix it in a separate water bottle to ensure you don't leave any.

3) Get 40 to 60 grams of liquid carbs post-workout. Dextrose powder, a commercial sports drink, or two pieces of fruit will work. If your protein source is milk, you may not need extra carbs. Check your labels.

******

Try to make sure your post-workout shake has no fat in it (under 5 grams is okay). Fat just gets in the way at that time. *Essential fatty acid* supplements or fish oils shouldn't be taken then. They can reduce inflammation at a time you might want *some* (to provoke muscle growth). Also, **do not consume extra multi-vitamins, minerals or anti-oxidants post-workout**.

Research shows these block *too much damage*, and as a result, your body might not overcompensate, i.e. grow.

******

And so there you have it, the post-workout shake. If you have it, and time it correctly, you will be perfectly covered for the next few hours. You will read recommendations about having another shake after an hour, but this is *not* necessary if you get this first one correct.

By the time you hit your next meal (3 to 5 hours later) the need for speed is reduced, and regular solid food (a balance of proteins, carbs and hitch-hiker fats) will do just fine.

Before we move on, here's a reminder of how much protein you need generally, and how it's divided between post-workout and your other 3 meals. Remember, your main goals are:

- **getting 40 grams post-workout**
- **hitting your daily target before you hit the sack**

If you can roughly balance the remaining protein between all 3 meals (4 on days you don't train), even better.

Bodyweight (lbs) and protein spacing for *Super Swole*

110	**88g a day**	40g post-workout & 48g from other meals
120	**96g a day**	40g post-workout & 56g from other meals
130	**104g a day**	40g post-workout & 64g from other meals
140	**112g a day**	40g post-workout & 72g from other meals
150	**120g a day**	40g post-workout & 80g from other meals
160	**128g a day**	40g post-workout & 88g from other meals
170	**136g a day**	40g post-workout & 96g from other meals
180	**144g a day**	40g post-workout & 104g from other meals
190	**152g a day**	40g post-workout & 112g from other meals
200	**160g a day**	40g post-workout & 120g from other meals

Bodyweight (kg) and protein spacing for *Super Swole*

50	**90g a day**	40g post-workout & 50g from other meals
55	**99g a day**	40g post-workout & 59g from other meals
60	**108g a day**	40g post-workout & 68g from other meals
65	**117g a day**	40g post-workout & 77g from other meals
70	**126g a day**	40g post-workout & 86g from other meals
75	**135g a day**	40g post-workout & 95g from other meals
80	**144g a day**	40g post-workout & 104g from other meals
85	**153g a day**	40g post-workout & 113g from other meals
90	**162g a day**	40g post-workout & 122g from other meals

BRO VS PRO

bro

✕ you don't have to eat anything special after working out
✕ the post-workout shake is old science & not relevant now
✕ only protein / only carbs / only water is what you need

pro

✓ get 40g of liquid protein within 15 to 30 minutes of training
✓ add 40 to 60g of liquid carbs to this meal
✓ add 5 to 6g of creatine monohydrate

SECTION 3:
EVERYTHING ELSE

ONE-SIDED VICTORY

If you work out in a gym long enough, you'll see all sorts of weird training. Eventually, you might notice someone who does many one-sided movements. You could assume they're an athlete, or training like that because they're injured. You could be right. But you could also be looking at someone who is actually advanced. One-sided training is a powerful way to make gains, even on *Super Swole*. Scientists call it **unilateral** training, as opposed to regular two-handed stuff, known technically as **bilateral** training. The athletes of years gone by didn't have a name for it, but often, it was most of their routine.

Take Eugen Sandow, the strongman born in 1867, who regularly used one-sided movements to train, and also to demonstrate his strength. This was a guy who at 5'9" and 190, could bent press over 300 pounds. What's a bent press? It's picking up a barbell with <u>one</u> hand, somehow hoisting it up to shoulder level, and then pressing it *fully* overhead. 300 pounds, or 140kg in the metric system, is h-e-a-v-y, even today. So, what's so cool about one-sided training?

DISPROPORTIONATE STRENGTH

Sandow instinctively realized that whenever you use *one* side of the body at a time, it can deliver more than just 50% of both-sided strength.

In a barbell curl for example, you might be able to get 6 reps with 70 pounds. But if you curl one dumbbell, you could get 6 reps of 45, over half of the two-handed curl. By using one side, the body can send slightly more of an electrical impulse through your nerves, resulting in more muscle fibers being fired up, and hence, more strength.

Over time, this increased strength can improve gains. This pattern of muscle "recruitment" makes sense, as many of our most natural activities rely on using *individual* sides.

MIND-MUSCLE CONNECTION

For most guys who workout, this is the greatest benefit of one-sided training. **By concentrating on one side a time, the extra electrical impulse generates a super hard contraction**. Combined with the fact you're literally focusing your attention on one area of the body, your sensation of working that area is heightened. For many body parts, especially the hard to "feel" ones, this could <u>massively</u> increase gains.

Ironically, most people's experience of one-sided training is limited to the biceps or triceps, two muscle groups which already have a strong mind-muscle connection. The real big boys, legs, chest and back, rarely get one-sided special attention. I'm not suggesting you change *all* your training to one-sided, but if you find yourself with a weak mind-muscle connection, doing some unilateral movements makes sense.

SYMMETRY

By using one-sided movements, you'll quickly even out any imbalances between the left and right sides of your body. It's surprising how quick this happens, proving that imbalances aren't generally made by nature, but are caused by nurture, i.e. us favoring one side over the other. This happens due to the naturally lazy habits we form in a modern environment. For guys who work out, symmetry is mainly a visual concern. But eventually, poor symmetry *can* lead to an injury. Ironically, injury is most likely to happen *during* a two-sided movement. Which neatly leads us on to the final reason for going one-sided.

INJURY PREVENTION

As just mentioned, training one-sided evens out any symmetry problems between left and right sides of the body. If you *never* attempt to correct these imbalances, injuries creep up. If you're a music lover, think how frustrating it is to hear tunes with the sound louder in one speaker. Well, your body is more sophisticated than any stereo, and leaving it like that is not music to its ears.

Common examples of imbalance injuries are the shoulders hurting on bench press, and pain in the lower spine after heavy squats (which you might not feel on one side, but it usually is). Injuries in lopsided pulling movements, e.g. pulldowns or pull-ups, are rare, mainly because our biceps and other elbow flexors compensate quickly (an ancient survival mechanism; handy if you're chased off a cliff by a saber-tooth tiger and need to hang on for a while). For example, it's common to see someone with a strong right bicep and weak right lat. If you're left-handed or left dominant, this could be the other way round.

Back to squatting and pressing movements. If *they* become too asymmetrical, you risk serious injury. This will either happen *acutely*, that's in a single moment, e.g. when benching you push way too hard on one side, and that shoulder goes. Or it will happen *chronically*, that's over time, e.g. in the bench example, gradually your dominant shoulder joint starts to get sore and eventually deteriorate, perhaps even needing surgery. If you're lucky, you might hear some grinding and popping noises from the joint. Always listen to your body's warning bells.

******

Not all one-sided movements are sensible. You have to think them through. Ask yourself a few questions before you commit to a one-sided movement:

1) Do I really *need* it?
2) Is it a *good* movement? (some are rubbish)
3) Is it *safe*?

For example, a one-sided leg press performed carefully, is great for balancing out your left to right power balance. But a one-legged squat, even though an amazing movement, is just too much of a risk for someone seeking symmetry. The forces on the spine, especially for anyone who has been unbalanced for a while, could easily create *new* problems.

This too-much too-soon difficulty usually puts people off one-sided movements. They forever think those exercises are just too fiddly to get benefits from. In fact, it's just because they're too far-gone in terms of skill. It only takes a well-chosen movement and a couple of workouts to feel like an expert.

It's important that you get clear about this one-sided stuff. I am not talking about standing on a stability ball, and trying to curl. This is often called "functional training", which is a silly phrase considering **all training performs a function**.

Don't be put off by skinny jeans/genes guys doing weird stuff, and assume they're ambassadors of one-sided training. They're not.

Here are some good one-side movements to fire up your imagination and give you a starting point should you ever need it:

LEGS

Single side leg press
Play about to find the optimal safe position for legs and hips.

Single side leg curl
Standing is especially good.

Single side leg extension
It should be called *knee extension*, and used <u>rarely</u>, due to forces on the patellar tendon; only use last 60 degrees of movement.

LATS

Single side pulldown
Use a "stirrup" handle, or a fabric / nylon loop.

Single side row
Aka: dumbbell row; just proving you might do one-sided already!

Single side cable row
Rarely seen, but effective for building mind-muscle connection.

CHEST

Single side floor press
Fantastic movement, but find a safe place to do it.

Single side dumbbell bench press
Also great, needs a fairly low bench to be safe.

Single side cable cross
Powerful isolation movement rarely seen, useful for sports.

******

If you are going to use a one-sided movement, you can easily cut your rest times to 1 minute. By the time you finish one side, you've already started rest time for that portion, and hence usually need less on the clock.

BRO VS PRO

bro

- ✗   one-sided movements are for weirdoes
- ✗   one-sided movements can't build mass
- ✗   one-sided movements don't do jack

pro

- ✓   one-sided movements are for smart trainees
- ✓   one-sided movements enhance mind-muscle connection
- ✓   one-sided movements could even be useful for you

PRE-WORKOUT

Since the year 2000, a previously unheard of supplement category started to make waves in the supplement industry. The **pre-workout**. These refer to any product taken up to one hour before your session. They're intended to boost workout intensity. Notice the word *intensity*. It's a difficult word to pin down, and that's why supplement makers love it. They use similar words including *primed*, *pumped*, *focused* and *energized*. These words aren't just difficult to pin down, they're deliberately non-scientific. That is: they're impossible to measure.

I FEEL SOMETHING

Now before I hate on them too much, it's undeniable that pre-workouts do *something*. They will make your ears tingle, your heart race, and sometimes, you'll feel a bit *funny*. Bros love this stuff! It feels like a secret, a one-up on your competition.

Most pre-workouts start with one key ingredient: **caffeine**. Caffeine, to its credit, is well-researched. It has positive effects, so much so, that too much of it in your blood will get you an Olympic ban. Lose your gold medal because of Starbucks? Yep.

Caffeine stimulates adrenaline release. And adrenaline is our main *fight-or-flight* chemical. It increases heart rate and temperature, diverts blood to the inner body, helps accelerate stored fat usage, and boosts the excitation of nerves. This last point can increase force production (strength).

So far, so good. Without doubt, even if you don't train, you're likely to hit caffeine on a daily basis. The problem is that very quickly, the body gets used to it. To get a powerful effect, you need to use caffeine rarely.

Research shows that one hit of caffeine doesn't affect hormones, but every caffeine source *after* the first one *raises* cortisol. That's the body's main stress hormone. And that's a problem.

In normal amounts, cortisol is fine, even useful. It helps raise blood sugar at key times, increases digestion, and can improve short-term memory. But in excess, it has a wide variety of downsides, some especially bad for gains. It can increase the rate at which you break down muscle, and it makes the muscle you have *less* sensitive to insulin. Remember, insulin is a storage hormone. After your workout, you want sensitive muscles in order that they readily absorb protein and carbs. So, too much caffeine = too much cortisol = too little absorption. There's a little section on caffeine at the end of the chapter if you want to know more, and maybe get off it.

BETA MALE

The second most common pre-workout ingredient today is beta-alanine. It's an amino acid (a part of a protein) used by the body to make another protein called *carnosine*. Carnosine levels in muscle are linked with the ability to perform "work" of slightly extended duration. By building up high levels of muscle carnosine, research shows you will develop less fatigue in activities that last between 60 seconds and 240 seconds (no, not *that*). If you work hard - between 1 and 4 minutes - you tend to build up lots of lactic acid. This is because you're not getting enough oxygen in, compared to how hard you're working. As a result, you burn stored carbs (glycogen). Whenever you burn glycogen, lactic acid comes along for the ride. Curiously, animals like deep-sea fish and dogs have super high levels of carnosine. It's as though they were made for that particular burst of energy.

In humans hitting the weights, you will actually be under tension for much less time than this. But if you train at a fast pace for long enough, lactic acid levels stay high even between sets.

And it's with those kinds of workouts that beta alanine seems to improve "muscular endurance". In theory, if you get more reps in the bag, you could indirectly improve muscle growth. A few studies have shown this, but the effect is small.

Placing beta alanine in a pre-workout *sounds* scientific, but like creatine, its effects are mainly due to building up high levels from one workout to another. Therefore, it might be smarter to take beta-alanine *after* a workout, and build up high levels for your next one. Remember, if caffeine is too high, cortisol will be high, and you might not absorb much of anything.

There is also a possibility that by preventing lactic acid levels from building up, you are *reducing* growth. Some research shows that lactic acid triggers growth hormone. Growth hormone itself is a trigger for other powerful hormones (such as IGF-1 and testosterone). Therefore, dampening down the burn with beta alanine could be a long-term gains' blocker. If endurance is your thing, beta alanine makes more sense. But even then, endurance athletes need to adapt in their mitochondria (cell components which generate energy). For getting swole, I'd give beta alanine the run around.

THE CHAIN GANG

Branch-chain amino acids (BCAAs) are three amino acids - *leucine, isoleucine* and *valine* - linked to stimulating muscle growth and boosting endurance in long events. They've been bubbling around forever. In the last few years they've resurfaced, and often appear in pre-workouts. And actually, that's not a bad idea. One of the branch chains, leucine, has been shown to increase mTOR, the growth factor known to kick-start gains.

Unfortunately, some pre-workouts give such a tiny dose of the branch chains, I can't justify the expense or effort. What about a specific BCAA supplement as a pre-workout?

Sure, great idea. It's called protein! As mentioned much earlier, getting 20 grams of protein one hour before you train is a smart thing. With 20 grams of protein in total, it's *highly* likely you will have enough of the branch chains to stimulate your body's muscle-building machinery.

BEWARE OF THE SINGLE MAN

Some supplement companies have grabbed the positive research on leucine and taken it to promote *just* leucine. This often means large doses of *just* leucine in their products. Nature is not stupid, and although leucine alone can get things moving, it needs its fellow amino buddies to work properly. Taking *one* individual amino acid can quickly produce strange physical and mental problems, as single aminos do not occur in nature's foodstuffs. Amino acids normally get through your blood-brain barrier in the right proportions by sharing a kind of raft to cross it. Your body only allows a certain amount and proportion of aminos on each raft. This stops potentially big amino "bullies" from having a raft all to themselves, and causing chaos. When you isolate *one* amino - something that never happens naturally - it gets the whole raft and massively raises brain levels of *that* particular amino. This can be sickening, sleep inducing, or downright dangerous depending on the amino in question.

Even having the three BCAAs might be a bad idea. And if you think this is all fear mongering, know that regardless, **studies reveal whole proteins cause the greatest anabolic effect**. Stick to those, and don't be seduced by a single or trio of desperate aminos.

This seems like a good time to mention a particular sales tactic.

B.S.™

If you ever see what's called a "proprietary blend", or spot a trademark symbol ™ on a label, avoid it. This is where a manufacturer wants to *hide* what's really in a product, and makes it seem more scientific than it is. It's a technique used by the beauty industry. By using a "blend", they can hide the exact proportions of a product, including the tiny amounts of the expensive ingredient you thought you were getting.

The trademark symbol is often next to made up buzzwords which make consumers think they're in good hands. Instead, you're in a good businessman's hands. Using the example of BCAAs, you might find someone advertise a BCAA blend of "3 grams". Research has shown that 2 to 3 grams of leucine might stimulate muscle growth. In our mythical company's blend, there might only be 1 gram of leucine, and 1 each of isoleucine and valine. This formula would not be effective, and unfortunately, you'd never suspect a thing. Why would a company do this? Because wholesalers who make leucine know it's in demand, and put the price up. Supplement companies then make less profit, unless they *suggest* the product has lots of leucine in it via a "proprietary blend" of ingredients.

Don't let companies B.S. you with science. The only powerful blend is the one *you* make by selecting individual ingredients, which you then chuck in your shaker. Do that, and you'll know *exactly* what's gone into it.

JUST SAY N.O.

Two supplements, citrulline and arginine are the other main ingredients in today's pre-workouts. Both are amino acids designed to increase **nitric oxide** production in the body.

Nitric oxide is a compound made in the body that helps the inside of your arteries expand. This area - the *endothelium* - is the part of your pipes that control blood flow through them.

In theory, by raising the body's nitric oxide production, you could increase nutrient delivery, and of course, *the pump*. Practical use of these products confirms that. The effects vary between people for unknown reasons. What's lesser known about excess nitric oxide production, is that it could increase oxidation in the brain. That is <u>never</u> ideal for long-term brain health. There aren't any studies long enough to assess the dangers of artificially raising Nitric Oxide (NO).

Another problem is that bizarrely, despite an enhanced pump in some people, it can often *reduce* the mind-muscle connection. This is because the training emphasis shifts to purely pumping, i.e. chasing the burn. While some lactic acid triggering is natural, it's not supposed to be the *main* focus.

There are natural nitric oxide boosters such as beetroot, but it's worth knowing that your workout itself boosts NO nicely. A solid pump is best achieved by intense mind-muscle connection, and adequate intramuscular carbs, i.e. glycogen. When you store carbs inside your muscles, you also store water (2.7 grams of water for every 1 gram of carbs). A muscle full of water and carbs pumps easily. This is why some people instinctively prefer training later in the day, when a combination of higher temperature, blood flow, and muscles *full* of carbs ensure a great feeling. If you rely on a natural pump, there will be no chemical come-down (which happens with pre-workouts). This is nature's intended deplete and restore cycle. Just say NO to N.O.

INNOCENT VITAMINS

Finally, many pre-workouts now contain large amounts of individual vitamins, minerals, or both.

While there's little wrong with these in general, having them *pre-workout* could damage gains. Emerging research is showing that anti-oxidants and similar nutrients can block the damage of resistance training so effectively, there's less reason for your body to adapt, i.e. less reason for it to grow. If you had to do high-volume *cardio* training, you might want to reduce damage, literally so you could run most days of the week.

Companies include these nutrients because some research *associates* higher levels of them with endurance, strength or recovery. This is a massive re-telling of the truth. These factors help *over time*, and *not* just before a workout. For example, B-vitamins help you extract energy from carbs, but that doesn't mean popping some with your *Gatorade* will turbocharge it. It takes a longer-term approach to ensure that. So, in your pre-workout *and* post-workout meals, avoid large doses of added vitamins and minerals. Take them at other times.

Pre-workouts are like a foreman shouting at workers in the factory. Although they try to respond by working harder, they've actually got limits determined by other things (muscle glycogen, blood sugar levels, and general recovery from good sleep and rest between workouts). Just shouting (pre-workouts) won't cut it.

******

There are many more supplements and pre-workout ingredients on the market, but just stick with the basics.

You already have to work on hitting those daily protein totals. Before we go, here's a quick section for those who are already on pre-workouts.

BREAKING BAD (HABITS)

If you are already addicted to pre-workouts, the quicker you break the cycle, physically and mentally, the better.

Relying on them is risky. You end up feeling you can't perform *without* them, which undermines general self-confidence. In addition, large doses of caffeine - the powerhouse of pre-workouts - cause mood swings and heart palpitations. It's no wonder really, as caffeine in nature is actually an *insecticide* (it scares off, irritates and eventually kills insects).

The most common problem when stopping pre-workouts is *caffeine withdrawal*. A caffeine withdrawal headache *hurts*. This happens because caffeine normally *dehydrates* the **middle cerebral artery** of your brain. When you stop caffeine, the water floods back through it, putting pressure on pain receptors.

A small dose of caffeine - around 25 mg - can stop a caffeine withdrawal headache. It does this by slightly dehydrating the middle cerebral artery once more, relieving the pressure.

But, if you use just this low amount for 3 to 4 days - *and then stop* - you're less likely to trigger a headache and other problems (e.g. sudden tiredness).

If you're in real pain regardless of a gradual withdrawal, seek medical attention.

******

A nice cup of tea or coffee is one of life's pleasures. Use its caffeine for a once-daily jolt, and you'll be fine. If this is pre-workout, and it makes you feel great, even better. But don't get more crazy than that. Being super-high in energy is no good if the downside is getting super-low. **Level is best.**

BRO VS PRO

bro

- ✗ pre-workouts are essential for great workouts
- ✗ trademarked blends help you beat the competition
- ✗ getting a pump is what a workout's all about

pro

- ✓ relying on pre-workouts eventually reduces confidence
- ✓ use low-dose caffeine to break addictions if necessary
- ✓ the best pre-workout is protein, food and proper recovery

HOWDY PARTNER

In this section we discuss training partners, whether you need one, and how to benefit from them if that's how you roll. It might seem like a personal topic that doesn't need discussion, but the choice to use one or not potentially affects many areas of your development. Let's answer the most basic question right now.

DO I NEED A TRAINING PARTNER?

No. And, you don't need a personal trainer either. Some guys and girls only hire them because they like someone to talk with. This is slack. Still, I'd rather they kept them instead of not hitting the gym at all. While mentioning that, let's start with the positives.

TRAINING PARTNER BENEFITS

Motivation for consistency

The first positive is the one we just touched upon. Working out with a partner makes *some* people more consistent. It could be for practical reasons, like getting a ride to the gym, or it could be psychological, i.e. working out with someone motivates you to keep schedule. If that's you, perhaps because you're new to the gym and a little bit awestruck, then it makes sense to have a friendly face around you.

Secondly, a training partner can increase safety. The simplest way is by giving you a spot (easy on the bench press, awkward on a squat). Being spotted gives many guys confidence to find their limits. In a true beginner, this can be very important as limits often **suddenly** present themselves. Being stuck under a heavy load is potentially life threatening (not to mention embarrassing). With time, you'll become experienced enough to work very close to the limit *without* needing a safety net.

A training partner can also boost long-term safety by checking out your technique. For example, it's handy to know if you push much higher on one side during a bench press, or if your knees and hips move unevenly during squats. Again - *with time* - you should be able to feel these things yourself.

So, those are the main benefits of a training partner, increased motivation and more safety. But what about the drawbacks?

TRAINING PARTNER DRAWBACKS

I firmly believe that training partner problems *outweigh* their benefits, especially after you've trained for a while. Here we go.

Damaged mind-muscle connection

This is without doubt the main problem of training with people. Visit any gym, and you will see groups of guys pushing each other during their sessions.

It may look like *YouTube* motivation, but your muscles don't care. They care about what's going on *inside*, and that's dominated by your mind-muscle connection.

The moment you react to outside stimulation, i.e. a partner's voice, or even just the general pressure of them watching, there's a **loss of concentration**.   This means a **loss of mind-muscle connection**. In a nutshell, you're <u>out</u> of the zone.

A reminder: it's mind-muscle connection that helps you *hit muscles you want to hit*, and it's the quality of that connection which allows you to *hit them hard*.   All this translates into more growth and faster growth.   In certain muscles - like the lats - a loss of mind-muscle connection ruins gains because of the intense concentration needed to *feel* them.   Being screamed at to do more pull-ups might sound cool, but you're just notching up reps and probably not hitting the target much.   This works for *Crossfit* types, but their mentality isn't on our page.

Also, using excess weight - *for you* - just because a training partner is stronger, or perhaps because you can't be bothered to change the weight, also ruins mind-muscle connection.   This is an extremely common and sad sight in the gym.   Sad?   Yes, it is sad, because it literally defies the beautiful aspect of weights, in that they can be perfectly tailored to *you*.   The original scientific name for weights was *progressive resistance training*.   Progression can happen without *always* adding weight, and sometimes without even adding reps.   But progression <u>cannot</u> occur if you keep breaking your mind-muscle connection.

A training partner who constantly pushes you, or affects your concentration at crucial times during a set, is robbing you of gains.

You need to extract all the gains out of a particular weight before adding more.   You must *master* that weight.   Training partners make you feel like the weight's slave.

Injury through excess reps or weight

Interestingly, breaking the mind-muscle connection also increases your risk of injury. It's ridiculous when a training partner says "come on, two more", as there's no real way they can make that judgment call <u>accurately</u>. Your ability to hit clean reps is a highly elaborate process, affected by *internal* factors like ATP, nerve stimulation, lactic acid and glycogen. Your pal in a tank top cannot assess those! More reps just for the sake of them *isn't* the goal. Reps much beyond your natural **clean form** limit increases the chance of overuse injuries like tendonitis. They could even push you to a muscle tear. Always - *always* - strive to maximize the mind-muscle connection. If your technique gets sloppy just because you're being barked at, an injury becomes likely. And worst of all, it would be *your* fault. Get reps to the beat of your own drum.

When mind-muscle connection is at a *peak*, injury risk is near *zero*.

Getting out of sync

When you're training with a partner, there is a natural tendency to match their rhythm and synchronize, i.e. match their pace. No two people - including *identical* twins - have the same energy or recovery level from the previous workout.

This means there will always be an imbalance between training partners, and if you match someone else's pace and effort, you'll be out of sync with *yourself*. In some cases this leads to physical and mental exhaustion, especially if you go out too fast. At other times you might be going too slowly, especially if your partner's sick, tired, chatting jive or moaning about their day.

When you're out of sync, you can't have an optimal workout that's based on *your* mood and muscle.

Exercise selection

This actually covers all the points we just made. If a training partner is dominant, and suggests using exercises that aren't suited to *you* ("dude, you gotta try this"), *you* might end up injured, bored, muscularly not stimulated (no mind-muscle connection), or worst of all, resentful.

Again, this is a common sight in gyms, with training partners certain they're in possession of a mass-gaining "secret". The reality is some exercises are not suited to everyone. Telling a guy who's 6'3" to barbell squat might not be ideal, especially if he leans too far forward, putting his spine at risk. Or, telling someone with tight shoulders to do heavy dumbbell flyes is effectively telling them to find a chiropractor.

When you train *without* a partner, you're less likely to pick and stick with obviously damaging exercises. Therefore, you're more likely to choose enjoyable and productive ones.

And for those who keep quoting *Pumping Iron*, stating that Arnold trained with Franco or others, I've got news for you. He didn't. He acted for the camera (it had a script), and for the vast majority of his training, Arnold trained alone. Today's bodybuilding pros appear to have training coaches, but in fact, they're mainly on hand to offer advice on "supplementation".

*****

So, with the assault on training partners over, is there anything more to say? Yes. There is a great training partner compromise.

Train alongside friends, but not *with* them.

Being in a gym "alone" can feel boring and demotivating, especially if the gym is your refuge from a horrible outside world. In which case, it's nice to know that when you stride out onto the gym floor, there's support in the form of a friendly face. There is nothing un-macho about this. Humans *are* pack animals. Liking and getting on with others is actually the essence of being human.

So you could either go to a gym with a buddy, and do your own thing, or just get friendly with those who train around the same time. Either way, you'll get the mental boost of being with like-minded people, as opposed to sometimes thinking, "What am I doing here?". You'll also be able to get a spot if necessary. Don't make that a habit though, because it could suggest you're training too heavy, and stepping out of the mind-muscle connection sweet spot. Obviously you need a smart buddy to understand these concepts. In an ideal scenario, you can get on with *your* workout, and yet still be social. For athletes training in a particular sport, training with a coach may be necessary. But if getting *Super Swole* is your priority, consider training without one.

BRO VS PRO

bro

- ✕ without a training partner bro, you're not serious
- ✕ you need a training partner to get a spot on each set
- ✕ Arnold had Franco and others

pro

- ✓ training by yourself improves mind-muscle connection
- ✓ training alongside friends makes solo training optimal
- ✓ Arnold posed with Franco and others, but trained alone!

GYM ETIQUETTE

For anyone who lifts in a gym, this section is important. You might think it's pointless to talk about how you behave. Don't worry, it's not a list of rules. Your gym will probably do those. And here's my quick take on what should be the important ones:

- **Put your weights away** (*all of them*)
- **Don't talk to someone during their set** (*even a friend*)
- **Respect people's space during a set** (*anywhere near them*)

This mini section is actually about the three most...

FREQUENTLY ASKED QUESTIONS

There are 3 questions you're likely to hear in a gym. They are:

- Are you going to be long?
- How many sets have you got left?
- Can I jump in?

Depending on how experienced you are, and how you handle social interaction generally, these questions might:

- confuse you
- annoy you
- intimidate you

If you are intimidated, it's understandable. But think logically: no one will start a fight in an enclosed public space if you answer them "incorrectly". So, how should you deal with them? Let's start with the first couple.

Are you going to be long? / How many sets have you got left?

The correct answer is:

Tell the truth.

Just tell whoever is asking the number of sets you're going to do.

You do not have to explain <u>what</u> you're doing. It's your workout, and no one has the right to judge it.

Seriously dude, you're having a workout, not sending the country to war (i.e. detailed explanations are <u>not</u> required!). Some clowns will see you working on equipment they want to use, and might selfishly be tempted to approach you *while* you work. If a clown does this, here's the drill:

If someone interrupts your set, don't react.

Concentrate, close your eyes, and continue.

If they persist before you're finished, ignore.

We instinctively understand that interrupting others is rude, especially if they're doing something physical. If someone is selfish and ignores that instinct, you can rightfully ignore *them* until your set it completed.

Occasionally, people will watch from a distance and assume you've been on a piece of equipment for a while. As such, they'll expect you to finish up soon. If they approach when you've actually just done your warm-up set, they may be surprised to learn how many you have left. In fact, they may take it personally. Unfortunately, many people are egocentric, and this doesn't change inside a gym (it often gets worse). So, what's the correct answer in such tricky situations?

Be honest. Be straight. That's it.

If someone raises an eyebrow about anything you do in the gym, don't react. If they *directly* ask why you're doing something, keep it short (e.g. "It's just what I do" / "It works for me" / "I just like it"). Hopefully they realize you're sincere, and go somewhere else for a bit. **Never fall for intimidation tactics, i.e. someone sitting or standing next to you until you finish. Always keep to your planned pace**.

Alternatively, they might ask the following question:

Can I jump in with you?

It's your <u>choice</u>. Whatever you do, it's okay. There's no legal obligation to instantly share gym equipment!

Generally it's a nice thing to do, and it keeps the gym friendly.

If you like training at a set pace, i.e. you use a stopwatch or your phone's countdown timer, let them know. You could work around it, or so could they.

Most people who interrupt your workout will be keen to not upset *you*, the person helping *them* out.

Now, even if you are a nice guy and let someone work in with you, don't let them put you off your stride, i.e. don't do your sets too quickly.

When letting someone work in, stick to your normal pace.

If necessary, let them go again, i.e. suggest they do another set before you do your next one. Extra rest is smarter than rushing.

GROUP INTIMIDATION

Sometimes, two or three guys might come over and ask you those three questions. This can happen at busy times, like evenings, or when happy-go-lucky *weekend warrior* types often train, e.g. Saturday mornings. Here's the first thing to know:

Don't let a group of guys intimidate you.

Simply being outnumbered does not reduce your right to use a piece of equipment.

If someone clowns around close to you during your set (clowns feel safer with fellow clowns), or drops a heavy dipping belt next to you:

Stay strong.

This is perhaps your **one life**, and you have a right to live it without another grown-up naked baby pushing you. Again, be real: tell the truth, act it too. If they ask to work in, and you think they might *really* slow your sets down, just say. It's unlikely though, as groups always giggle and rush through their sets (conversely, advanced trainees train alone). The same guidelines about not letting others interrupt apply here. Close your eyes, re-focus, and finish your set normally. Set the pace, never follow it.

DO UNTO OTHERS

With all of this said, I hope you apply the same common sense to others if you need to get on something. Although a full-body routine will probably have a desired order of exercises, it's fine to mix up the order sometimes. Yes, even if it causes a few of your numbers to drop for *that* session. As long as you train hard, and push hard on your last set, growth will be stimulated.

So there it is. Be cool in the gym, and try to realize that everyone's on a mission. Whatever that mission is - it's important to them - and we can all relate to that. And even though gyms themselves can have annoying rules, try not to get banned.

I know you're upset about not being allowed to squat barefoot like Arnold. I'm sure he'd still have done okay in a pair of *Nikes*.

BRO VS PRO

bro

- × forget etiquette, hell yeah!
- × I got here first, so it's my space!
- × My training's more important than *them*, so get off that!

pro

- ✓ everyone's on a mission, so it's smart to respect choice
- ✓ don't be bullied off equipment by a guy or a group
- ✓ treat others like you'd like to be treated in the gym

WEIGHING UP YOUR OPTIONS

There are many ways to measure progress. Let's bust through them and see what your options are.

SCALES

Obviously, there's the basic weighing scale. If you're someone who happens to always maintain roughly the same level of body fat, then using scales has some use. If you go up, you're probably adding muscle. And if you go down, you're probably losing. Probably.

But even then, there are changes *inside* the body, like gaining or losing **visceral fat**, a fat stored deeper behind your midsection. This is not to be confused with fat just under the skin, called **subcutaneous fat**. In many people, their subcutaneous fat doesn't change much when they start a program, i.e. their abs don't look like they're changing. But inside, they're often losing lots of visceral fat. That's great for general health and maximizing testosterone production.

If you're going to use scales, and most can't resist, use these guidelines:

- weigh yourself once per week on a fixed day
- weigh yourself after the same routine (e.g. after the bathroom)
- buy your own scales and don't let anyone else use them
- put them on a hard floor which doesn't wobble
- never use the gym's scales

The last point is important. On average, at least 50 different people per day will use locker room scales. That's like using private scales once a week - for a year - <u>in one day</u>. Even the best scales can't handle it. You need accuracy.

MECHANICAL OR DIGITAL?

Digital tech has come far, and is easiest to read (especially in small weight jumps), so I'd head that way. Pick the best you can afford, but don't buy gimmicks. Go mid-range, and ignore features you'll never use, e.g. BMI or data storage. There's pen and paper for that, and actually, who ever forgets?

BODY FAT SCALES

The science behind measuring body fat via scales is much better today. Still, it's not perfect. They work by shooting electricity through your feet, up your leg, over your groin (it doesn't hurt), and back down the other leg. The amount of resistance the machine finds helps it estimate what you're made of. Fat and muscle have a different density, and hence different resistance.

The problem with these scales is that they estimate your *entire* fat and muscle proportion based on your *legs*. On average, that might work. But you're not Average Joe! Some guys have naturally skinny legs compared to their upper body. This might make their body fat look low (and possibly, their muscle mass too high). Some guys might have the reverse of this.

For overall accuracy, these BIA scales (bio-electrical impedance analysis), aren't useful. There are hand-held devices that measure upper body fatness and muscularity (by shooting electric from one fingertip to another).

In theory, if you used both hand and foot devices, you'd get a decent picture of where you were. Is it worth it? I'd say no.

MEASURING TAPE

Oh come on, every guy measures! And this includes the classic upper arm measurement. Does it help? It's fun, but measuring too frequently is just a recipe for driving yourself mad. If you're running *Super Swole*, it's cool to measure once at the beginning and end of the program. **Get a fiberglass measuring tape**. They don't stretch or shrink. A workman's metal tape is fiddly.

If you want to measure, do it at 4 key places:

- **upper arm**
- **upper thigh**
- **around the chest**
- **waist**

These four will give you a rough idea of progress, and they're classic barriers to break through, e.g. surpassing 16" arms or shrinking your waist below 32". Remember, bone structures and muscle attachments vary, so measurements can't perfectly predict how you'll be changing. Solid 16" guns on a 5'10" guy will look awesome. But on someone who is 6'3", their impact is less impressive. And for those guys who moan because they have tiny wrists, don't worry. It's *easier* for you to look great, especially when the shirt comes off. Muscle flares wildly from small joints.

If you must measure, do it infrequently. Generally, 4 times a year is enough to keep an eye on progress. Any more is overkill.

CALIPERS

Skinfold calipers do what they say, i.e. they measure folds of skin in certain places, and use formulas to convert the numbers into fat and muscle percentages. They can be accurate in a controlled environment like a university lab. And without doubt, **to use calipers properly, you need someone to help you**. That's not just because some places are awkward to reach, but because if you did it yourself you'd be less consistent and maybe less honest. You can kid others if you like, but never kid yourself.

DEXA SCANS

In an ideal world, you'd get a DEXA scan to find out how much muscle and fat you have to start. Then, go back later to see what's changed. Because science fears giving you too much radiation (DEXAs use X-ray), you can't get scans too frequently. In fact radiation from DEXA is low, but providers realize that users are interested in precision, and precision gets addictive. It's unlikely that you could get scans every 6 weeks. The lowest waiting period is usually every 8.

DEXA scans are highly accurate. Modern scanners give you data on not just muscle, fat and bone, but also let you know how much visceral fat you have. And, they break the body down into sections and sides. It's useful - and sometimes a bit shocking - to compare your right arm to your left, or your upper body to your lower.

For example, people often discover that their right leg contains 2 pounds *more* muscle than their left. If you get access to this data, it can encourage you to train carefully, i.e. with dumbbells.

One thing DEXA can't do right now, is calculate how much fat you have *in* your muscles. This is called **endomysial fat**.

Science is divided about it, with some saying it's useful for strength in big lifts or endurance, while others suggesting it means your body is incorrectly depositing fat. For now, there's nothing the average person can do to measure it, so let it slide.

DEXA is an amazing technology, and I encourage you - at least once in your life - to get a scan.

Prices are dropping, with local universities often being the cheapest. Having said that, finding those who will do them is often tricky. Your best bet is to go straight to a private testing facility. All Olympic athletes and most professional sportsmen now use DEXA, realizing the benefits are both interesting and useful.

FIVE PERCENT JIVE

One warning: be ready for the DEXA truth to shock you. It's common to hear locker room talk about being "5% body fat".

Being 10% body fat or under is very, very lean. Less than 1 in 10,000 people are this. And most can't hold it.

I have seen people with good abs around 20% fat. At a genuine sub 10, it actually *hurts* to sit on wooden chairs. Faces look skeleton-like, with razor-sharp cheekbones and a defined jaw line. Some of this makes a guy look more like a guy, but if you go too low, you could get the wrong kind of stares.

Some conservative health professionals say hormones like testosterone plummet if body fat is too low.

The data from ultra lean athletes, like Olympic gymnasts, generally show this isn't true. For your comparison, Olympic gymnasts *at* the Olympics are between 7 and 8% fat.

Problems with body fat mainly occur if it's too *high*.

In that case, testosterone isn't produced optimally, and what you do make doesn't work well. In women, low body fat can produce serious changes (e.g. periods stop). This happens at lower than 15% body fat, or in some, lower than 20%. Although those figures seem unfair, a woman under 20% will look very lean. Surprisingly, some "supermodels" with low bodyweight have been found to have *high body fat*. Effectively, they are small in size, but have not much muscle. Training with weights would improve their health dramatically. Not that you care!

OBSESSION

While measuring how much you change can feel scientific and smart, it can also take away the fun. And believe me, fun is important to sustain long-term improvements. During *Super Swole* or any training, it's okay to *not* measure anything. You'll already be measuring success by seeing your weights go up, or even just by seeing yourself in the mirror. These things can be a great guide. It's obvious when training is going well, and over time, remember that anyone with a decent program *will* improve.

If you think you have the potential for becoming obsessed, *kill it now*, and just get on with having fun in the gym. Fun keeps you moving in the right direction.

BRO VS PRO

bro

- ✗   weigh every day bro, or you won't know what's happening
- ✗   breaking the 16/17/18/19/20" arm barrier is crucial
- ✗   you're fat bro unless you're 5% body fat

pro

- ✓   use DEXA if you want accurate measurements
- ✓   more weight in the gym can be a good guide in itself
- ✓   genuine 10% body fat (20% for women) is shockingly lean

LET'S BREAK IT DOWN

Although the body can push hard for a long time, it's smart - every so often - to give it a break. As in, **a complete rest from training, lasting 1 whole week**. This achieves 3 things simultaneously:

- you give potential injuries a chance to heal
- you mentally "pause", which then boosts motivation
- you see your training and life balance in perspective

INJURIES

Although a week off from the gym isn't enough time to heal a serious injury, it is enough time for minor ones to get a head start. Curiously, many people find that *during* a period of time-off, injuries begin to show themselves. In many ways this makes no sense. Except it does. When you're in the gym, you're high on adrenaline and other natural painkillers produced by working out itself. These endorphins (**endogenous**, produced within + **morphins**, painkillers resembling morphine) are powerful and switch off pain. When you stop training - i.e. when you stop self-medicating on endorphins - pains slowly reveal themselves.

Don't panic if this happens, because you've been given a chance to shift things around. It could require a change of exercise, a change of technique, or a backing off in weight. This last possibility is especially true if your ego has been driving your workouts. In sport science, backing off is called a **de-load**.

If you are going to de-load, make it meaningful and cut back to 50 to 75% of your normal poundages. Above that intensity, nothing may heal. Effectively, you're just having a bad workout.

If you discover an injury, stick to 75% max until things improve. It may take a couple of weeks. Be patient.

If you have any sense of being overtrained, a week off is exactly what your muscle tissue and overall system needs. Try to do *nothing* physical during the week. Some sport scientists encourage "active rest", a concept that allows you to perform "light activities" you wouldn't normally consider, e.g. play tennis, or swimming. How quaint. And how utterly illogical! The concept only came about because kind sport scientists couldn't deal with their moaning athlete's demands to do more! *Active rest* is potentially dangerous and certainly defies the point of resting in the first place. My advice: **do nothing**. Enjoy it, do some binge viewing on *Amazon* or *Netflix*, pig out. By doing nothing, you'll be doing everything that's good about a break.

PSYCHOLOGICAL PAUSE

The great thing about habit is the buzz of self-discipline and control. The bad thing about habit, is boredom. And don't underestimate boredom. It's a factor that can persuade people to change their careers (or partners, or both, *usually just before New Year's Eve or Valentine's Day*).

What everyone finds after a solid week off is that they're *raring* to go once their break is over. Seven days away energizes in the way no pre-workout supplement ever can.

LIFE / TRAINING BALANCE

During the week off, naturally you will either miss the gym or be relieved about the break. If you're balanced already, it will be a bit of both. Regardless, the time away presents an opportunity to value how important training is in your life.

Even if you can say with certainty - *I love training* - a little week off will reinforce it in your subconscious. You may also face things that your training has been disrupting, i.e. non gym stuff. Again, this is a golden opportunity to see the bigger picture, and shift things around to improve your overall *work / play* balance.

I hope you're now convinced to take breaks. The only question remains, how often should you do them? Well, on regular programs, the usual recommendation for this tactic (called *deconditioning* by scientists), is 7 to 10 days off every 12 weeks. On **this** program, which has a greater frequency in terms of muscle stimulation, I suggest this:

Take 1 week off from training, after 6 weeks of going all out.

Some of you might think it's way too much, and fear you'll shrink. Trust me, you won't. At the very least, when using an intense *Super Swole* routine, take a week off every 2 months. Research shows you will not dramatically lose your gains. Drug using athletes who stop using steroids *as* they stop training, do lose size quickly. This is because they're going from ultra-high testosterone to zero (the body's negative feedback loop shuts down hormones when you "shop elsewhere"). Your testosterone will generally be stable (natural testosterone only has slight seasonal variations, peaking slightly from April to October).

Muscle memory is a non-scientific but still correct term for the way humans re-build muscle fast.

Muscle cells which aren't stimulated may shrink slightly, but they don't actually disappear. Simply restart training to send them some electricity, and they will jump back to life.

Be cool: **take a break every 6 to 8 weeks. Your body and mind will thank you for it.**

BRO VS PRO

bro

- × never rest bro, just kill it 24/7
- × if you take time off, you're just wimping out
- × you lose all your gains the minute you stop

pro

- ✓ taking a week off heals injuries & informs you about problems
- ✓ taking a week off helps you re-calibrate the *work/play* balance
- ✓ taking a week off re-energizes your training upon your return

PUTTING IT ALL TOGETHER

If you are genuinely new to training, you might have found parts of this book intimidating. That's to be expected with any new challenge. Pretty soon you will become more relaxed, and more of an *expert*. And that's important, because training with weights is mainly a solo activity. You have to do all the thinking, planning, and of course, doing. But it *is* worth it, as only you gets all the glory.

To achieve success, you will probably have to shift a few things around in your life. The way you eat, the way you sleep, and perhaps even the way you think in general. You don't need to do this all at once, even if this book is promoted as a 6 week plan. I'd rather you *gradually* improve all these areas bit by bit - no matter how long it takes - and then be set up for the rest of your training life.

Because social media and the internet is so influential, there will be times where you question this plan, your genes, or everything in general. This is normal, and it's actually smart to be a bit skeptical. Having said this, you will make great gains if you initially trust someone to guide you (i.e. me!). Flip-flopping from routine to routine is all too common, and it's a destroyer of gains. *Super Swole* may appear old-fashioned, but it's worth remembering how old-fashioned we are as a species.

The first step for most people is to get on the right routine with the right frequency. A full-body workout is the way to go. If you have the guts to think independently, you won't believe the hype about it only being useful for beginners. Find out what works in terms of frequency by simply paying attention to your body's signals. "Listen" out for what feels right. *Feels* sounds wishy-washy, but we live a feelings based life. You need to discover the best schedule for your particular genes, lifestyle, and mentality.

As cool as working out is, it's for a reason, and that reason usually is out of the gym itself. Find balance.

The next step, once you've got the training down, including all the tips on mind-muscle connection, is to master your food. Well, master your palate. It's fine to enjoy food, in fact it's a goal in itself, but you must be aware of what you're doing in order to distance yourself from *Average Joe*. You don't have to become neurotic and cause chaos amongst friends when choosing a restaurant. Just be mindful that you need a bit more protein than most, and you're better served by 4 balanced meals a day instead of 3 or 10 (seriously, most people pass something with calories past their lips 10 times a day).

And finally - after a while - when you have food and training ticking over nicely, experiment with some advanced techniques. Try some one-sided training, take a week off every so often and come back like a beast, perhaps using some new moves. Keep the mind-muscle connection high at all times, and I assure you, you'll make progress faster than you thought possible. In many ways, your success starts *before* you get into the gym, with a decision to give it your <u>honest</u> best. If you've struggled to gain before, don't assume that's you for life. Genes vary, but we also share a common physiology. You will progress if you follow the guidelines in this book.

Once you get beyond 6 weeks, there is absolutely no reason to suddenly do another program. The temptation to try new things is almost a human trait, so control it, and instead keep pushing on the basics. Most people do them very badly. I know that if you've read this far, you are not most people.

Right. Don't **P-A-N-I-C**, it *will* make sense! Seriously.

Get in the gym.

Let's finish with a double sized *bro vs pro*.

BRO VS PRO

bro

- × dude, this is some old-fashioned stuff
- × do splits, and definitely hit chest on Mondays
- × work every muscle from every angle to look like a pro
- × go for the burn and chase the pump on every set
- × forget protein, just bulk up with everything in the kitchen
- × it's all about weight baby, so get it up at all costs

pro

- ✓ use full-body workouts every other day to every third day
- ✓ use a high volume, hitting 3 to 6 sets per muscle group
- ✓ do 4 to 10 reps, getting heavier each set, failing on the last
- ✓ eat 4 meals a day, roughly spaced apart, balanced in macros
- ✓ get 20g of protein before, and 40g after each workout
- ✓ focus on mind-muscle connection at all times & you will grow

USEFUL LINKS

It's always a risk to hook people up with strangers, and website recommendations are no different. But there are a couple - well, three - which are quite good. Use them as a starting point if you're looking for more. Here they are:

examine.com

This deals with supplements and general nutrition. It's impartial, i.e. not paid for by supplement companies. Instead, the emphasis is on research. If something works, this site will explain why, and neatly arrange all the studies for you to look at. As nutrition and supplementation continuously evolve, this book cannot keep up (though the basics will never change). I advise you to go there from time to time, especially if you hear some broscience bigging up a new "discovery". Look before you leap.

exrx.net

This is an exercise physiology site, with excellent coverage of most major exercises. Going through the site takes a while, but like *Wikipedia*, it's hyperlinked, allowing you to quickly jump from one related idea to another. For example, if you click on "pec major", it will flag up the functions of the muscle, and generate lists of exercises. It's a handy reference, and especially useful if you're up for changing parts of your routine. You'll get some real insider knowledge on muscle function, which helps you avoid broscience easily.

This combines the first and second sites, plus a bit of research news, into a neat and clickable info source. The site digs up the latest research on nutrition, supplementation, training, psychology and general health, then puts it into language anyone can understand. It really is fascinating. If you want to keep up with on-trend developments, and still be aware of existing ideas, this is where to head. The writing is simple, making research enjoyable. Beware, you may become addicted.

******

There are some decent *YouTube* fitness channels to fire up enthusiasm, and also cover developments as they happen. Of course, it's all about personalities and whether they click with you. Even if that doesn't happen, you're finding out what and who you do like.

Athlean X

This channel, run by physical therapist Jeff Cavaliere, heavily talks about exercises themselves. Although Jeff promotes a paid program, his free stuff covers lots of ground. His understanding of proper technique is excellent, having been a therapist for the *New York Mets* baseball team. If there's an effective way to do something, or a dangerous way, Jeff will *show* you the difference. As he records many of his videos with his shirt off, you can see that he both talks the talk, and walks the walk.

Strength Camp

This channel, run by Elliot Hulse, is a solid mix of training talk, some nutrition, and a whole lot of motivation. It's this last point that sets Elliot apart from many of his equally knowledgeable peers. While his training advice is generally sound, it's his sensible yet gung-ho attitude which many find inspiring. No joke, getting swole is fun, but it also takes an attitude shift, and Elliot's one of the best guys to help you do that.

Bios3 Training

This channel, run by former competitive bodybuilder Jerry Ward, is a friendly yet fired-up place for training, nutrition and drug talk. The last area - drugs - is important, because knowledge of it puts it in perspective. Making drugs a taboo subject serves no one. In fact, it tends to exaggerate their benefits and reduce their drawbacks. And often, advice about training applies to whether you're on drugs or not at all. Jerry tells it how it is with honesty, and that's both refreshing and informative.

THE LAST REP

Well done for reaching the end of this book. Seriously. In today's world, we all tend to be looking down at our phones, and skipping past the scenery that could inform our journey. You've made an intelligent move to better your knowledge, and even that attitude puts you in the top 1% of humans. But when you put this book down and start taking action, you will almost certainly face people who call your determination *obsessed*. They might be buddies at the gym, people you work with, a girlfriend, a boyfriend, or even your family.

F**K THEM!

I had to emphasize *the importance of being yourself*. Yes I know, you've heard and seen that sentence e-n-d-l-e-s-s times. I'll say it differently:

We're all planes trying to take off. Don't let anyone distract you. If you do, you could run out of tarmac. You are the pilot. Take charge today. Go <u>full-throttle</u>.

Finally, I'd like you to remember this:

Having a great body is a very noble goal.

It's not shallow at all, but instead respects the amazing machine we've been given.

Even if you workout *just for muscle*, training will bring you better physical health and an inner confidence that will make you a happy person to be around. And happiness spreads. No one can argue with spreading happiness.

So, get out of here - *get out there* - and attack your plan with *everything* you've got. If this is your one life, make it just the way you want.

Stay swole.

JACK ARMSTRONG

February 29, 2016

Venice, California

* * * * *

#superswole

www.ingramcontent.com/pod-product-compliance
Lightning Source LLC
Chambersburg PA
CBHW070801280326
41934CB00012B/3014